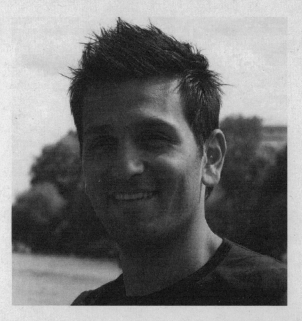

Joe is a former England professional basketball player, with over 10 years experience in fitness and health training and coaching. Joe founded the Fitness Boutique in 2005 and has trained a vast range of clients from competition-ready athletes to busy mums wanting to shed baby weight. Joe and the Fitness Boutique team are also retained by a number of celebrities, international royalty and several leading film production houses to ready film stars for major − and often demanding − roles.

The Red Carpet Workout

Joe Fournier

headline

First published in 2009
by HEADLINE PUBLISHING GROUP

1

Cataloguing in Publication Data is available from the British Library

978 0 7553 1868 1

Typeset in Bodoni BE Regular by Avon DataSet Ltd,
Bidford on Avon, Warwickshire

Printed and bound in Great Britain by
Clays Ltd, St Ives plc

Headline's policy is to use papers that are natural, renewable and
recyclable products and made from wood grown in sustainable forests.
The logging and manufacturing processes are expected to conform to the
environmental regulations of the country of origin.

HEADLINE PUBLISHING GROUP
An Hachette Livre UK Company
338 Euston Road
London NW1 3BH

www.headline.co.uk
www.hachettelivre.co.uk
www.theredcarpetworkout.co.uk

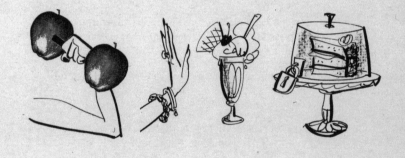

Contents

Chapter 1   So who is this guy and what can   1
             he do for me?

Chapter 2   Why will this plan work?   27

Chapter 3   The plan. If you're only going   51
             to read 18 pages, make it these

Chapter 4   What to expect, week by week   71

Chapter 5   Drinking and the fun stuff. Oh,   85
             and how to stop making excuses . . .

Chapter 6   From Pret to Pizza Express . . .   103
             The essential eating-out guide

Chapter 7   Everything you need to know   119
             about exercise – and some
             fascinating facts

Chapter 8   What on earth does that mean?   139
             Why does that happen? And is
             that *really* true?

Chapter 9   And when you're finished . . .   161
             The essential maintenance bit

Chapter 10   Case study: Sarah's been there   177
             and done it – here's her story

Chapter 11   For those of you who don't use   195
             your oven to store shoes . . .
             here are some recipes

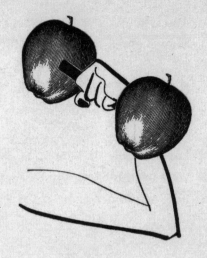

Chapter 1

So who is this guy and what can he do for me?

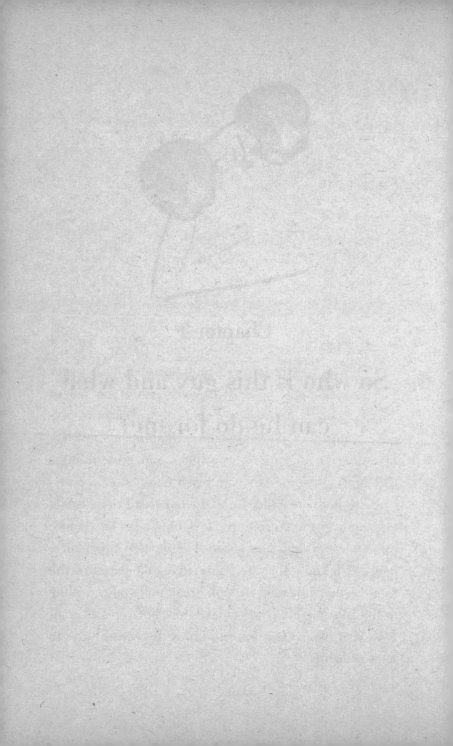

About Me

If I had to sum myself up in a few words, I'd say I'm a celebrity personal trainer, a former professional basketball player and a big fan of pizza and champagne. There, I said it. I'm not a fitness angel, I don't spend every minute of my day dreaming about running machines and cross-trainers and I love going to bars with my friends.

I also hold my hands up to the fact that I'm naturally lazy and, given the choice, I wouldn't get up before midday every day. That's why I've devised this plan – because I know that it's more than likely you're the same as me. You want to look great, and you're willing to put in some effort to achieve that, but you still want to have a life, so you want to know the easiest ways to look amazing.

It was a revelation to me when I realized that I could be fit and still have fun, and it also made me see how completely ridiculous most of the 'miracle' diets on the market are. I don't believe that looking good means you have to eat tasteless food, spend half your life doing stomach crunches or never going out. That idea is dull, outdated and, ultimately, it doesn't work.

Looking and feeling good is all about doing things in moderation, which is why I can't understand why some fitness plans will happily put a total ban on booze and treats. That just leads to people feeling frustrated and wanting to give up before they've even begun.

That's where the Red Carpet Workout is different – you can follow the plan, lose weight and still go out and enjoy yourself. I'm not going to pretend that you don't have to put in any effort at all – of course you do – but you won't mind, because you're going to see quick results, learn a lot and really enjoy it.

Part of the reason I train is because, as a personal trainer, people expect me to look good. But it's also because *I* want to look good. I like to be able to take my shirt off on the beach and not worry about having overhang or moobs.

I've been a personal trainer for twelve years now, and I've trained some of the biggest stars in the world for anything from demanding movie roles to glamorous red-carpet events such as the Oscars. These people's livelihoods depend on them looking incredible, and I've whipped the best of them into shape in a matter of weeks.

I never reveal details of my celebrity clients (I'd be out of a job if I did!), but take it from me, if I were to show you before and after pictures of some of the people I've worked with, you'd be stunned at the difference a few weeks can make.

Over the years I've learnt which exercises I do and don't like, and I don't torture myself doing stuff I hate because I know I won't give 100 per cent. I think this is important for everyone, which is why I'd never tell you to go for a run if you hate running. In this book, I've given you a choice of exercises, so you can tailor the plan to suit you by finding something you actually like doing.

Around 80 per cent of my clients are female, so I know what works well for women when it comes to getting in shape. That's *why* I can promise you a body that's red-carpet ready in six weeks. All you've got to do now is buy yourself an amazing new dress to show it off.

How can the Red Carpet Workout make me look amazing?

The simple answer is: by ensuring that your body burns up more calories in a day than it takes in. This plan isn't about ridiculous juices, mung beans or doing a thousand press-ups before breakfast. It's about common sense. The plan is designed to give you a movie-star body in just six weeks, and that isn't just an empty promise. It won't always be easy, but it *will* be worth the effort.

The main foods I ask you to avoid are bread, pasta, cheese, nuts, potatoes, seeds, avocados, cream and sugar. You can still have these in moderation every now and again, but there are loads of other things you can enjoy. The plan isn't about depriving yourself of nice things to eat, it's just a case of finding food that does you good at the same time as tasting great!

It also gives you a bit of leeway to have fun and go out drinking if you want to. I know that, if a diet is too restrictive, the boredom soon sets in, so I'm giving you a 'wild card', which you can use when you want to take a break. I'm not stupid enough to think that you're going to want to spend the next six weeks without a drop of alcohol; it's something that is so much a part of our busy social and working lives that it's difficult to cut out, even if you want to. What's more important for me is finding that crucial balance between work and play.

It may be hard to believe, but celebs *don't* always look amazing. Trust me, as someone who has trained some of the world's top stars over the last few years, I've seen it with my own eyes. That perfect figure you see in films isn't the reality. Far from it! And even those people who are naturally blessed with great bodies have to look after them through diet and exercise.

Many celebrities relax in between films and events and let themselves go a little. Then, when they have a movie role coming up and they need to look incredible, or a big event is looming and they know they'll be under close scrutiny, they work their arses off to get into the best shape they can. That's where I come in. I'm often called upon to get someone red-carpet ready in as little as three weeks. This involves a strict diet and tons of exercise and dedication. But, believe me, it works. And that's how I know for sure that this plan will work for you.

Six weeks may not seem like a lot of time, but you'll be amazed at what you can achieve in that time. As well as losing some of that niggling excess weight (I'm guessing if you've bought this book you're hoping to drop some pounds!), you'll tone up, feel more confident and learn loads of fitness and diet secrets which you can integrate neatly into your everyday life. You can still eat out, you can still have fun at work do's and on nights out with friends, and you're not going to spend the entire time feeling as if you're torturing yourself. In fact, you'll feel so good when the weight starts to drop off that you'll find you're actually enjoying it.

I worked with one female celeb a couple of years ago who was desperate to get back into shape because several celeb mags had cruelly pointed that she'd put on a bit of weight. She had a big American awards do coming up, and she wanted to prove to people that she was back at her best.

She was still fairly slim, but she did have wobbly bits and, because she wasn't toned, she had overhang in several places where her clothes were cutting in. I concentrated on the main areas that would be seen in the dress she was going to wear to the awards ceremony and, by cutting down dramatically on carbs and working out as much as she could manage, when the time came for her to walk down the red carpet six weeks later, she was confident and happy and looked incredible. The following week she was back in the celeb mags for all the right reasons, and everyone was saying how amazing she looked.

We all want a quick fix, right? If you're anything like most women in the world, you'll have tried loads of different diets, gone through phases of exercising, and yet you're *still* trying to shift the weight that's stopping you getting into your skinny jeans. Well, those days are now over.

If you follow this diet and exercise plan to the letter, you will lose a couple of pounds a week and around ten to twelve pounds by the time the six weeks is up – if you have that much to lose, that is. (If you're already naturally slim and just looking to drop a few pounds, your weight loss is likely to be slower.) You'll also tone up. You'll see the difference in your body shape, both in and out of clothes.

The book is split into different sections, depending on how hard you want to work out and how much weight you have to lose. You can choose between the Lazy Girl, for those who are new to exercise and want to take it slowly, the Savvy Girl, for those who have exercised before or have more time on their hands, and the Fitness Queen, for those who really want to go for the burn and see super-fast results. Busy week ahead? Go Lazy. Want to ramp up the exercise and burn more pounds? Become a Fitness Queen. This plan works around you, for you.

Experts say that losing one to two pounds a week is a healthy rate of weight loss, and I agree. It's been proven time and time again that you're more likely to keep weight off if you lose at this rate. If you lose weight too fast, the chances are it will go straight back on again – and those niggling pounds will bring some friends with them. If you go on a diet that makes you lose weight ridiculously quickly, clearly, you won't have done it in a healthy way. All you will have done is to deprive your body, so, as soon as you start eating normally, it panics and retains weight to protect you in case you decide to do the same thing again. Welcome to the wonderful world of yo-yo dieting. Thankfully, this plan is the exact opposite.

Now, I could create a stupidly restrictive programme that you will hate by day two, but where's the sense in that? We all need something which is doable, as painless as possible and which gives lasting results, rather than a super-quick fix. That's what this book is *all* about, and that's why you'll love it.

In some ways, this programme *is* a quick fix, as it will get you results fast. But it's also a plan that can be followed long term. And, because you won't have hated every minute of it, like some diet or exercise regimes you've tried, and because you'll love seeing the incredible results you've achieved, the chances are that you'll *want* to stick with it. Once you discover forms of exercise you enjoy, you'll want to keep doing them, and it won't seem like a huge effort.

Imagine how good you'll feel when you've got loads more energy and you've finally done what you've been promising yourself you'll do for years – whether that's dropping a few dress sizes or just losing that bit of irritating excess weight that hangs over your waistband every time you sit down.

Just think, no more moaning to your friends about your muffin top, no more panicking about whether you'll still fit into last year's summer wardrobe. And no more being a food bore who skips from ridiculous diet to ridiculous diet without seeing any lasting results.

The fact that, with this plan, you'll be exercising *and* eating sensibly, which means that you're not going to wake up one day to find that the pounds have all piled back on without you even noticing.

And, because the plan is so simple, you can integrate it easily into your everyday life without even really thinking about it. It will soon become a way of life as opposed to a traditional 'diet', where you spend all day feeling deprived and miserable!

Once you've completed the programme, you can maintain your weight loss with an easy-to-follow toned-down version. You can follow the Lazy Girl workout (more of that later) and do fun types of exercise that you will enjoy, whether it's salsa dancing, boxercise or a few sets of star jumps before work (maybe don't do this one if you've just started dating someone new . . .).

The great thing is, it's not as if I'm saying that you have to go for a 10 km run every morning before work in order to keep from regaining the weight you have lost, just do some form of exercise a couple of days a week.

So, there it is. If you're dedicated, this programme *will* work for you. If you want to lose weight and look amazing but aren't willing to put in any kind of effort, then you may as well put this book down now, because there's no point in reading any further.

'I'm too busy' is the excuse that's used the most when it comes to people giving up on diet and exercise plans, but that won't wash with me. Buying or making healthy food takes the same amount of time as buying or making junk food, and that fourth hour you spend in front of the TV can be spent doing a form of exercise you really enjoy.

If looking fabulous were stupidly easy, we'd all be skipping out of the house looking like Giselle each morning. And, if you're one of those people who think that, one day, the extra weight you've been cursing for ages will just magically melt away without you even realizing it, think again. A good body is something that has to be worked at. I'm not pretending that the Red Carpet Workout is going to be a breeze – there are times when you'll want to give up and hot-foot it to the nearest bun shop, and I guarantee there will also be at least one moment when you'll wonder if it's all worth it. But, six weeks from now, when you slip into that fabulous new dress you've been hankering after, or you're showing off your new body on the beach, you'll look back and you'll know without a shadow of a doubt that it was worth every run, dance or cycle, and every piece of cake or pint of beer you've politely refused. And not only will you look better, you'll *feel* better, because, as well as your confidence going through the roof, you're going to feel a massive sense of achievement.

I've let myself go a bit – can I really get back on track?

Of course you can – just put in some work. Take it from me, pretty much everyone has to work to look good; they just don't like to admit it. I've trained celebrities that are perceived to be some of the best-looking people in the world, and I can promise you that they have had to put in a lot of effort in order to dazzle on the red carpet or look buff for their latest movie.

If I named names, I'd probably find myself without a single big name client, but I will tell you a few stories about people I've whipped into shape to prove to you that even celebrities aren't *born* perfect.

A couple of years ago, I trained an incredibly handsome and charismatic British actor – women literally swoon over him. He's made some really big movies with some of the most gorgeous female stars in the world.

His agent called me up and said that they needed me to get him back into shape, and give him a six-pack, all within just one month. I Googled some photos of him and thought, 'Well that's not exactly going to be hard.' He looked in pretty good shape from what I could see. What I didn't know was that, while he was between roles, he let himself go a bit. A lot of stars relax in between movies. They go home to their families, they get comfortable and they eat a lot and, before you know it, the weight has piled on.

Anyway, after I'd told the ladies who worked in my gym that this heartthrob was coming in, I came in the next day to find them in full make-up, literally bursting with excitement at the prospect of seeing this amazing actor.

While they were waiting for him to arrive, this guy walked in and said he was there to see me. The receptionist just looked at him all confused and said, 'I'll check if he's in, but I know that he's waiting for a client.' When he replied, 'Oh, that may be me, I'm—' she nearly fainted in shock, because he so didn't look anything like he usually does. He'd grown a big bushy beard, but what really shocked her were the pounds he'd piled on.

I went out to meet him and immediately wondered

how on earth I was going to get him lean and toned in a month. He was at least three stone overweight, and his face was really fat. Luckily, he was aware of it and said to me, 'I'm out of shape and overweight, but I'm willing to work hard to get results.' From the point of view of having to get incredible results in such a short time, he's the toughest celebrity I've ever had to train but, at the end of that six weeks, he had the six-pack. It meant we had to work out every day, twice a day, and follow the eating plan I outline later in this book, but he did it. And anyone who went to watch the film he'd got in shape for wouldn't have had a clue that, just a month before, he was so big he was virtually unrecognizable. That's dedication for you.

I have to say, actresses do tend to be much more motivated than actors, because being in the movies is such a competitive business and everyone is so image conscious. Look at how much weight Beyoncé lost when she was in *Dream Girls*. They know they have to look good to get the great roles, so they're much easier to train.

Many actresses who come to me are a bit 'soft' from having had time off, again usually between movie roles. They've relaxed a bit, stopped their usual exercise routine and put on a bit of weight.

I trained a very famous actress a while ago who has

a history off yo-yo dieting. When she came to see me, she was a bit overweight. Getting someone to lose weight can be relatively easy but, with her, we had to get her to lose it in the right way and to make her tone up because, to look good in a red-carpet dress, it's not just a question of dropping a few pounds, you also need to have the right posture and muscle definition.

Obviously, female celebrities don't want to look too muscly, but they always want their arms to look nice and lean, because they will be on show when they're in front of the paparazzi.

This particular actress was willing to put in the hours, she worked hard and, while she didn't want to look skinny, she went down a dress size, looked slim and healthy and achieved a weight that suited her. She's since remained the same weight and kept up the exercise, and she no longer yo-yo diets, which has made a big change to her life.

I also once trained a premiership footballer. We had two weeks to do some pre-season training, and I've never seen anyone push themselves so hard. The results he got in those two weeks were the most amazing I've ever seen, and he did it because he wanted it so badly. He wasn't trying to lose weight, but he lost three-quarters of a stone in that time and reduced his body fat hugely.

Everyone thinks that footballers spend a lot of their time partying and shopping and, yes, some of them do. But a lot of them are incredibly dedicated, and they work as hard as they do because they want to be the best. And it's the ones who are the best that train the most. It's as simple as that.

Lots of people who are generally considered to be beautiful have as many body issues as the rest of us. I worked with an A-list American actress who came to me convinced she had terrible bingo wings. She was in great shape, but I have to admit that, compared to the rest of her body, her arms weren't very toned.

She had a movie coming up and was going to be seen in skimpy outfits, so she wanted to look the best she possibly could. She was so conscious of her arms that she asked me to measure them when I arrived for the first day of training, and then every week throughout the six weeks I trained her. She wasn't worried about how much she weighed, and she didn't step on the scales once – for her, it was all about her arms.

When it was time for her to film the movie she was finally happy with them, and they did look totally different to when we first began. But it just goes to show that even those people we perceive to be perfect have hangups about their bodies.

I always say, if you're happy with yourself, great, stay

as you are. If you're not, you can change things. It's all about how you feel and what's right for you.

My final story here is probably the most bizarre and, again, it involved a very famous American actress (let's call her Actress A.) It was during the run-up to the Oscars a couple of years ago. When I arrived, she picked up a picture of another famous American actress (who we'll call Actress B), pointed to her body and said, 'I want to look like her.' As far as I was concerned, this seemed pretty odd, since they looked quite alike already.

Anyway, Actress A tried on her Oscar dress and, though there were a few lumps and bumps, I had eight weeks to get her looking like Actress B, and she was determined to achieve her goal. We worked out most days, and she followed a healthy diet and, when she tried on the dress eight weeks later, she looked incredible.

But what was even weirder was that, when the Oscars came around, it turned out that Actress B was wearing an almost identical dress to Actress A. Thanks to some hard work, though, at least Actress A looked every bit as good in hers, if not better.

The fact is, celebrities can't get away with eating or drinking whatever they want. It may look as if they're out partying most nights, drinking loads and yet never putting on weight. But that's because, if they are drinking a lot, they're also working out like crazy and watching their diets. Or they're pretending to drink a lot to boost their image.

I know one actor who's perceived to be a real bad boy and is always in the papers for being a big party guy, but I know for a fact that, if he goes out, he'll literally have one beer all night, because he doesn't want to put on weight. Sometimes you have to make a choice between partying hard and how you want your body to be. Like I said earlier, it's all about the balance . . .

How do I motivate myself?

Motivation tips
1) Remember that it's only six weeks out of your life. You won't have to be this strict for ever.

2) Remember that, after every low, there will be a high. So, if you feel terrible one day, the chances are you'll feel better the next day.

3) Remember how proud you're going to be of

> yourself at the end of six weeks, and how happy you'll be when you can fit back into your old jeans.
>
> 4) If you're feeling as if you're on the verge of giving up, use your wild card and treat yourself. Just don't let it kick off a downward spiral.
>
> 5) Stick the worst photo you can find of yourself on the fridge and look at it every time you wonder what you're doing it for.

The best way to motivate yourself is to set goals. Right now, six weeks may seem like a long time to stick to the plan, so it's all about keeping in mind what you want to achieve.

So many people are stuck in that rut where they hate exercise, but they're also desperate to lose a bit of weight. Whether it's dropping five dress sizes or just that difficult last half a stone that really doesn't seem to want to shift, we've all got our own reasons for wanting to drop some pounds.

If you're anything like a lot of the people I've trained over the years, you've probably already tried every diet going. You've ditched booze for a few weeks, joined a gym that you've been to maybe four times in the last year. Yet you still seem to find yourself back at square one. That's why it's time for a different approach – one that you can stick to and which will give you results. And one that *won't* take over your entire life.

The best way to stay on any new diet and exercise programme is to have your goals set out firmly in your mind. What do you want to achieve from this plan? Do you want to tone up? Get a better bum? Or just get fitter? Nearly all of the celebrities who come to me have an end goal in sight, and it's that that makes them work so hard. One actress says she mentally pictures herself in her awards dress every time she feels like quitting, and that spurs her on.

We've given you a chart to fill which you can download from the website (www.theredcarpetworkout.co.uk), so start thinking now about what you want the Red Carpet Workout to do for you, and then write down your aims. You can write as much or as little info as you want, and then stick it on your fridge or by your desk at work. That way you'll always be able to refer to it at those moments when you're tempted to give up and dive into a family pack of salt and vinegar crisps and a bottle of rosé.

We all have different reasons for exercising, and it's very important to know what yours are. A lady came to me recently for personal training. She was around a size 20 and, when I asked her what she was hoping to get out of being trained, I admit I expected her to say that she wanted to lose weight. Instead, she told me that she was very happy with her body the way it was and simply wanted to improve her fitness levels so she didn't get out of breath when she was walking up lots of flights of steps or running to catch a train. She came to see me knowing exactly what she wanted to achieve, and that made it easy, because she focused on what she wanted and, together, we achieved it. If you don't have a goal, you can be working for eternity without really getting to where you want to go.

If you get on a treadmill not knowing how long you want to run for, at what speed and what gradient, you'll get bored after a couple of minutes. But if you say to yourself that you're going to go for ten minutes – no matter how tough it is – you will keep going for that amount of time because you've set yourself a challenge.

If you decide to go for a run around the block, you'll do it. If you just go out for a run and don't have an aim, you'll probably stop halfway down the street because you don't have an end goal in sight. Whenever I'm training people, if they're on a piece of timed equipment, they always ask how long they've got left, because then they can mentally pace themselves, which really helps them to stay focused.

Also, think about why you really want to lose weight. Are you getting married? Have you got a big birthday coming up? Or do you want to look good in a bikini for an upcoming holiday? It's great to have something to aim towards.

Who am I doing this for?

Another really important thing to remember is that you have to be doing this plan for *you*. When people come to me for training, I always ask them, 'Why are you here? Do you want to be here, or has your husband or boyfriend bought you some sessions and pushed you into coming?' If that's the case, then people are always far more likely to give up.

A perfect example is a celebrity who I trained for a magazine photo shoot last year. She was really up for following the plan and seemed to be working hard in her sessions, and then the magazine shoot fell through. She turned round and said to me, 'Why am I still training? I'm not doing the shoot any more, so there's no point. And if they do decide to do the shoot again, they'll airbrush me anyway.' And that was the last I saw of her.

The problem was that she wasn't doing it for *her*, she was doing it because she was being paid to and, once that motivation fell by the wayside, so did her enthusiasm. It's a real shame, because she was already starting to look great but, once the money incentive was gone, she lost all interest.

I always say that, if you're happy the way you are and you don't want to go from a size 16 to a 12, then that's totally up to you. If you're happy, stay happy. You need to *want* to lose weight or tone up for *you*. However, by picking up this book you're basically saying that you want to change things about your body – either a little or a lot. And, with this plan, you can make a *huge* difference in just six weeks. That's why it's easy to stick to and so different to everything else out there. So, let's cut those excuses and get on with it. The sooner you start, the sooner you'll see fantastic results.

A friend in need . . .

If you feel as if you may need extra motivation while doing the Red Carpet Workout, the best thing you can do is rope in a friend to do it with you. Why? Because, when you don't want to exercise, there's always going to be someone there to motivate you and, by the same token, when they don't want to go out on that run they promised they would, you can spur them on.

It also makes things become slightly competitive (in a good way), and competition brings the best out in us. Why else do you think people panic when summer starts looming and they know they have to go and sit on the beach alongside loads of other semi-naked people? It's all about vanity. We want to look better than the person on the sun lounger next to us. Fact. Of course, I'm not suggesting you sabotage your friend's exercise just so you can 'win', but trying to match them as they get into better and better shape is a brilliant way of keeping motivated.

More importantly, having a fitness buddy also makes exercise more fun. You can have a gossip while you're working out, and it also takes away the worry of going to a new gym or exercise class on your own, which lots of people can get a bit nervous about.

The biggest secret when selecting a fitness partner is to find someone who has pretty much the same level of fitness as you. If you choose someone who is much fitter than you, rather than her spurring you on, you may feel de-motivated because you can't keep up with her. And, if you have a partner who is way below your fitness level, you may not work as hard because you'll feel as if you should exercise at their level.

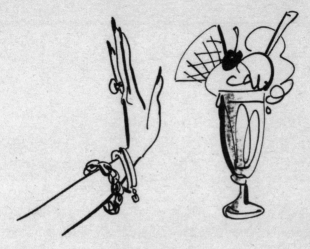

Chapter 2

Why will this plan work?

As I said before, the Red Carpet Workout will teach you how to burn more calories than you take in. It really is that simple. I've created an eating plan that's easy to follow and can fit in around your life. There's no point in telling you to live on things like fruit juice or fry-ups for six weeks, because those kinds of diets are too extreme and aren't manageable in people's everyday lives.

Of course, there are restrictions on what you can eat if you want to lose weight, and I'm not going to lie about the fact that there are quite a few on this plan. But it's all about listening to your body and retraining yourself to want to eat more healthily. It's not the kind of finger-wagging plan that will make you panic. It's designed to fit around you and your busy lifestyle, and you can even drink alcohol on it – though, as we'll see, this doesn't give you a licence to go out and get drunk every night!

It's no secret that diets won't work if they're not doable. In fact, many people give up on them after only a matter of days because it's just not viable to fit those kind of eating plans around your day-to-day life.

It's not as if you can take six weeks off work just to do the plan. And, even if you could, you'd be bored within a couple of weeks and would probably give up altogether. With the Red Carpet Workout, you don't have to wave goodbye to your social life, and you won't feel miserable while you're doing it, as people often do on stricter regimes.

Look at it this way. If I told you to run a marathon tomorrow, it's very unlikely you'd be able to do it (unless you've been training for a very long time). But if I told you to run 500 metres, you probably could do it without too much effort.

If I said to you that you had to eat rocket for breakfast, iceberg lettuce for lunch and water for dinner, how many days are you going to keep that up for? One? Two? Three at the most? Then you'd go and eat a pizza. But if I told you to just cut out a few of the things that you'd normally eat, you wouldn't be half as tempted to give up.

There are juicing diets that promise you you'll lose seven pounds in a week. Unsurprisingly, you *will* lose a lot of weight, since you're not actually eating any food.

But are you going to sustain that weight loss? No. Are you going to ask for just a glass of juice every time you go out for dinner? No. Are you going to take your juicing machine into a meeting with you and start whipping one up when you want a snack? No. And we all know what happens when you start eating normally again. The weight just piles back on.

Those kind of regimes just aren't realistic. This plan is. It's gradual, and it will keep you on the right track, because you don't have to starve yourself at a party if they're not serving tofu skewers – you just create a balance with what you eat. Remember that health is all about balance. If you ate chocolate every day of your life and never brushed your teeth, the chances are that your teeth would fall out. But if you ate chocolate *and* brushed your teeth, the chances are they would be fine. It's the same with your body: you can eat and drink and have treats, but you have to do something to counter-balance it – exercise.

The Red Carpet Workout is all about doing things that are achievable, and healthy eating and taking regular exercise *are* achievable wherever you are and whatever you're doing. And, before you start worrying, I'm not going to be suggesting that you take a plastic bag of mung beans into work with you to nibble on during your morning break or that you run a marathon before breakfast every morning. Far from it: you'll be eating delicious, wholesome food, with some treats thrown in (including the odd glass of champagne) and discovering that exercise isn't about killing yourself – it could even turn out to be something you enjoy . . .

What if I feel like giving up on day one?

Then you won't be alone. But bear in mind that the first few days are always the toughest on any kind of diet or exercise regime, so don't panic. As I've said before, I'm not going to pretend that you can do this without hard work and, if you haven't broken sweat for a while, it's going to be tough to begin with. (This is another reason that I'm all about moderation and balance – imagine how you'd feel facing up to going on a run if you had to live on carrot juice alone!)

I see plenty of clients who want to give up after their first training session.

I had one female client who hadn't exercised for ten years before she came to me and, as she admitted herself, she was very lazy. At first, she kept making excuses not to come along to her sessions, then I pointed out that, not only was she wasting money but that she was just delaying the inevitable. She knew she wasn't going to be happy until she got herself in better shape, so I explained to her that it was better to do it sooner rather than later. That way, she could reap the benefits for longer. She totally agreed, started coming to see me regularly and, within a month, she could see real results. She was also shocked to find that she was actually enjoying coming along to the sessions. One of the reasons my clients come to me (and keep coming back) is because they know I'll be around to help get them through these difficulties early on. I guarantee that.

Now, I won't be there personally to give you a kick up the arse when you need it, so you'll have to do that for yourself. But, you can refer back to the book any time you feel as if you're in danger of giving up, and it will help to get you back on track and be reminded of your goals.

You've got to trust that this plan is going to work. AND IT WILL. Read the next few pages of the book whenever you feel like throwing in the towel and diving into a bag of sweets, and it should give you the motivation to keep going. And if you make a mistake or you fall off the food wagon, learn from it and move on. DON'T GIVE UP.

If you do falter every now and again, it's really important not to give yourself a hard time. I've been a personal trainer for twelve years now, and I've made mistakes and learnt a lot along the way. Making mistakes is the best way to learn, so think of them as a positive thing rather than beating yourself up about them.

When I first decided to get fit, I was desperate for results, so I lifted weights that were too heavy for me. I ended up with ridiculously painful shoulder muscles and a bad back, but I didn't mind because I could see that my arms were becoming more toned. I thought it was a case of 'no pain, no gain'. It wasn't until someone told me the correct way to lift weights that I realized I could still get great toned arms, without the pain. Now I know what weights suit me, but I spent a lot of money on massages in those first few months. The other thing I learnt from this is that exercise doesn't need to be about punishing yourself. What I always tell my clients is that the best thing they can do is find something they enjoy. Just because something is fun, it doesn't mean it's not doing you any good. And vice versa.

I've tried so many diets and exercise plans in the past and given up. Will this one *really* work?

Yes, because this plan is all about balance. There aren't tons of rules to follow, and you're not going to feel as if you're being tortured on a daily basis. I've trained enough women to know. For instance, you can drink on

Top five diet excuses

1) 'It's too expensive.' People say that healthy foods are more expensive than non-diet foods. That's not true, you just need to know where to look. If you buy a load of vegetables, you can make lots of different dishes for pennies. And you'll save lots of money when you're not out drinking every night.

2) 'I don't have time.' It takes just as long to buy something healthy as it takes to buy something that's bad for you!

3) 'Work gets in the way.' Even if you have to go to lots of work do's, you can make healthy choices.

4) 'I've got PMT.' Eating healthily will actually help your PMT, and it only lasts a few days, so you can't use that excuse for very long.

5) 'It doesn't taste good.' That's probably because you've been eating horrible 'diet' meals. There's plenty of delicious healthy food out there.

this programme, which is always a bonus in my book. Once or twice a week, depending on which plan you follow, you'll be able to enjoy vodka and champagne aplenty. All I ask is that you do a bit of exercise the following morning to balance things out.

It's so easy to get into bad habits – I've been there! – but I hope I'll be able to show you how to look at things from a fresh point of view. For instance, did I mention that I love pizza? I would eat it for every meal every day if I could, but I also like looking good, and there's no way I would get away with an all-pizza diet and not put on loads of weight. So I save pizzas for special occasions and, if I do overindulge and have pizza two days in a row, I'll be careful for a few days and make sure I exercise.

Another bad habit people get into is skipping meals altogether, which is not good. Our metabolism is like a log fire; it needs constant stoking and you do that by eating. If you get up and rush around, skip breakfast and then don't eat until midday, you haven't got your metabolism up and running and, obviously, it's vitally important that you do as this helps burn fat stores. This is why I would always advocate eating three meals a day (and snacks if you're still hungry). Nobody ever got into shape by starving themselves.

Why can't I just diet to look good?
Why do I have to exercise as well?

Sadly, diets on their own very rarely work. People often refer to them as a 'short-term fix', but they're not a fix, because they're not effective. The problem isn't really solved, it's just set to one side for a little while.

Maintenance is the secret to a happy, healthy body. That doesn't mean living like a saint or depriving yourself of anything nice, it just means moving around more and eating a healthy, balanced diet.

The basic truth is that, in order to get lasting results and for your body really to start looking better, you do need to exercise. Models are a great example of this. Everyone assumes that models are either just 'lucky' because they're naturally slim, or they don't eat anything. But the real top models have to work at it.

I've worked with several of them, and I can see immediately who puts in the hours in the gym and who doesn't. I was shocked when I first met one particular model, who I'd always thought was stunning. She was still very beautiful in the flesh but, when her friend put her arm around her, her hand was literally melting into the model's arm, she was so squashy there. Her arms were super-slim, but they didn't have even the slightest bit of muscle tone. And, even though she was tiny, she still wobbled here and there.

Some models *are* naturally slim, but they're not naturally toned and, in the world of modelling, only about 5 per cent of models worldwide actually do it as a full-time job. A lot of them do the odd job here and there, and then they have to supplement their income with other work. The big difference between models such as Naomi Campbell, Kate Moss, Gisele Bündchen, Heidi Klum and Elle Macpherson – models who get loads of work and last the distance – and all the other models is that they take it to another level. They train hard to make sure they look good and stay in shape. They may not want you to know it, but they work out like crazy, because they have to in order to stay looking perfect. They don't just turn up on shoots month after month and hope for the best.

You see some models walking down the catwalk and, yes, they're slim, but if you get up close to them, you can see that there's no muscle tone. I call that syndrome 'skinny fat'. Those girls are never going to be booked to front a large lingerie campaign. However, if you get up close to Naomi, you can see what amazing shape her body is in, and it will stay in good shape because she's done some serious work over the years. The girls who are making the most money are the girls who are in the gym every day.

It's the same with actors and actresses. Yes, some of these people were lucky in that they were born gorgeous, but that doesn't last for ever, and it takes work and it takes maintenance. Start thinking of yourself in the same way. You can look fabulous if you're happy to put in a bit of work.

Exercise also releases endorphins, which make you feel positive and better about yourself, and that's half the battle. When you feel good about yourself, you want to look good and treat your body well, which is what the Red Carpet Workout is all about. It's about being happy with yourself, whatever size and shape you are and want to be.

How do you keep fat off? (Get ready for some geeky stuff)

Exercise, exercise, exercise. The more lean muscle mass you have on your body, the more efficient it'll be at burning excess fat. The best way of building up your muscle mass is to exercise properly.

When you lose your muscle mass, it's a lot easier to gain fat. But, if you have a lot of lean muscle, it's much more difficult to put on fat. That's why, when people get chubby, they often then get fat. Then, when they get fat, they sometimes become obese.

Marathon runners do a kind of training called 'glycogen storing' which only burns fat. (Glycogen is what the fat stores in your body are converted into to give you energy.) They wake up very early in the morning, they don't eat breakfast, then they'll go for an hour's run. Normally, when you exercise, the first twenty minutes you do isn't spent burning fat, it's just burning the excess energy which is in your glycogen stores. So, if you run before you eat any food, you'll be breaking down fat stores, as opposed to glycogen, from the word go. When marathon runners do this training, their bodies become very efficient at burning fat.

When it comes to actually running a marathon, they eat a load of carbohydrates three days before, which lifts their carb stores very high, so that they're burning carbs as well as fat, which gives them more energy.

Like marathon runners, we need to train our bodies to burn fat as efficiently as possible and, needless to say, if we take in less fat and sugar, then that's what we'll do.

When people say they're losing weight, they're actually often losing muscle, because they crash diet and don't exercise, so the body eats into its muscles when it needs energy. As soon as they start eating normally again, the weight piles back on.

A person who has a lower percentage of body fat and a higher percentage of muscle will burn more calories during the day than someone who has a high percentage of body fat and little muscle, because their bodies have to work harder. Whatever way you look at it, exercise is good news.

I'm already pretty slim, so I reckon I can skip the exercise bit . . .

Not true. Think of yourself in the long term. If we were all skinny and toned, we would never bother to exercise. We'd all stay in bed snuggled up cuddling our pillow in the morning when we know we should be going for a run. But if we knew that, in ten years' time, we would pile on weight and feel unhappy, then we would be more likely to put our trainers on and get out there to ensure that wouldn't happen. It's a fact that it's easier to put on weight and harder to lose it as you get older, so it's almost as if it's damage limitation. Think about how many people say, 'I used to be so skinny. I could eat whatever I wanted and I never put on weight.' But that rarely lasts for ever. So much of staying healthy and looking good long term is about developing good habits while you're young.

A lady I know was a size 6 to 8 and won beauty-queen contests when she was a young girl. She's now a size 28, because she thought, 'I'm super-skinny, I've had two kids, and I haven't put on any weight, so I don't need to worry. I can eat croissants every day.' But, all of sudden, she started to put on weight, and it just kept going on.

She wasn't in very good shape and, because she hadn't exercised for years, her body wasn't working efficiently. It's so much more difficult to exercise yourself back to slimness once you've reached that level, which is why it's so important to try and stop the weight gaining process early. There'll inevitably come a point when you can't burn fat off like you used to be able to, but if you're exercising and in good shape you'll avoid becoming a victim of middle-age spread.

What are the other reasons why I should exercise? (When really I'd like to be in the pub)

The simple answer is: because of all the amazing benefits.

You won't be ill so often

Exercise helps to keep your immune system strong, so you get ill much less frequently. When you get run down, you get sick, but if your body is in good shape, it will be able to fight off infections.

How many people come back from holiday saying they've got 'Malia sickness' or the 'Marbella cold'. It's not because each foreign town has its own special illness, it's because, when people go to those places, they drink every day, they sleep very little and they get run down, so they pick up whatever is going around. It's the same with the 'city sickness' that affects people who work in London's City district. They work fifteen-hour days, they come home and have a bottle of wine and then they fall into bed and don't sleep properly. Your body can't cope under that kind of pressure unless it's in really good shape and, if you're not doing anything to counteract the effects of your bad lifestyle, you'll get ill over and over again. I haven't had to take antibiotics for years and years, and the trainers that work in my gym never call in sick, because we're all fit enough to fight off infections.

Exercise gives you a high

When you split up with someone, all you want to do is lie on the sofa and eat chocolate and drink wine. But, ultimately, you make yourself feel ten times worse. Yet if you pick yourself up and go and do some exercise, you'll feel so much better.

Okay, so it's not the easiest thing to do when all you want to do is sob, but the sweetest revenge would be to look amazing the next time you bump into your ex. Not only that, but exercise releases endorphins – the feel-good chemical – in your brain. The other thing that exercise is great for is giving you a real sense of achievement. The combination of all these benefits can be the perfect thing to help you get over a bad break-up quickly, but it will also keep your spirits up day to day.

Exercise makes you look good

We're all vain to a certain extent, and we all like to look good. Exercise makes you look good. It's as simple as that.

I'm French Italian, and we eat cheese – a *lot* – and plenty of carbs. But if I ate all of those foods all the time I wouldn't look lean and toned. And, from a purely vain point of view, I like having a six-pack, so that, when I go on the beach, all the girls fancy me.

In my opinion, this is the best by-product of exercise: looking hot. And it's not only a question of having an amazingly toned body. When you're exercising properly, you'll be expelling toxins from your body, so your skin and eyes will look far clearer and your hair will be glossy and shiny. And there's nothing us guys like more than girls with beautiful hair.

Just knowing that you're exercising makes you feel better about the way you look. And, when you feel good about yourself, it shows. You'll notice that curvy women who exercise are far happier with themselves than curvy women who don't. It doesn't matter what size you are, as long as you feel good about yourself, and exercise helps to give you that amazing feeling by helping to make you feel confident about your body.

You don't have to be a size zero to be sexy (in fact, like most men, I would argue that size zero isn't sexy anyway), you have to be happy inside and out, and exercise gives you a massive boost.

Exercising will save you time

Okay, so that may sound weird, but it's true. Exercise helps with your sleep patterns and, as you get fitter, you need less sleep, so you're able to get up earlier and get more done. And your quality of sleep will improve because you'll fall asleep more quickly and wake up feeling more refreshed.

Exercise will improve your work

Exercise helps you learn to be focused, and that spills over into your work. Think how much less work you get done when you've had a bit of a bender the evening before. You feel all over the place, you can't concentrate on anything and you waste hours staring at a screen or out of the window. But if you've been out on a big night and had a run, it will help to clear your head and you can see things more clearly. Even when you're not hungover, if you're exercising regularly, your energy and concentration levels will be greatly improved.

You'll also have to take fewer sick days, because you'll be getting ill much less, so your company will like you more or, if you're self-employed, you'll earn more money.

Exercise will help reduce cellulite

Exercise helps to break down the build-up of fat in pockets beneath the skin. There are a lot of theories about cellulite, and unfortunately some people will always have it, but you can reduce it massively through diet and exercise.

Everyone will get it eventually; it's about managing the process. And, if every part of your body looks toned and sexy, are you really going to worry if there's a stubborn bit of orange peel on your bottom?

Exercise will boost your confidence

A lot of businessmen feel way more confident after they've been to train with me. Suddenly, they're not afraid to take their suit jackets off in meetings, and they can tuck their shirts in without having to worry about their gut. Also, when your muscles are stronger, you stand up straighter and you look more confident.

Some people you notice the minute they walk into a room, and it's not because they're the best looking, it's because they move with confidence. Why do so many women fancy Mr Big from *Sex and the City*? He's not a bad-looking guy, but he's no Brad Pitt or Colin Farrell.

However, he is fit for his age, and he carries himself in such a confident way. He's the kind of guy who, in real life, would have a personal trainer and would work hard. He's powerful, and he's sexy, and that's what makes women notice him.

It's the same with the female cast of *Sex and the City*. None of them is classic model material, but they all look great, and they clearly work out to keep in shape. As a result, they feel good about themselves, and that shines through. They all carry themselves well, and they can all get away with wearing whatever they like because of how toned they are. They don't have perfect figures, and they've all probably got their own hang-ups, but they make the most of what they have and they work it.

How nice is it to wake up in the morning and not have to worry about what you're going to wear? You know that whatever you put on will look good, because your bum is in shape and your arms are toned, so you can sling on jeans and a vest top and look every bit as great as a woman who's wearing a ball gown.

No matter what you're wearing, if a man walks into a club, he'll notice the girl who's having fun and looks as if she's a laugh, as opposed to the girl who's sitting in the corner looking miserable. Not because she's necessarily the most attractive, but because she looks as if she's good fun to be around.

I trained a guy a while ago who was about five stone

overweight. He was in his fifties and had never had a girlfriend because he was so lacking in confidence. In fact, he was so shy it took him six months to build up the courage to ask me to train him. He worked hard and lost the weight and gained tons of confidence. Shortly afterwards, he was in a bar, saw a girl he liked and went up and asked her out. A year later, I went to their wedding. It wasn't that he couldn't have found a girlfriend before; he just didn't have the confidence. All that changed when he started to exercise.

Another former client of mine put on a lot of weight and went up to a size 20. She got very depressed because she couldn't meet anyone. She put in the work and, what she lost in weight, she gained in confidence. She's now a very happy, toned size 16 and has men queuing up because she doesn't shy away from guys any more.

When you find that confidence, it's amazing. I've met girls who are way out of my league, but I know that, when I feel good about myself, I'm more likely to be able to pull them. You will never see me out and about trying to meet girls around Christmas time, because that's when I'm out with my friends drinking beer, and my healthy eating regime dips a bit. While I may not look much different physically, I don't feel good about myself when I'm like that, so I don't feel as confident when it comes to speaking to women.

Exercise will improve your sex life

Sex is a lot less fun if you're doing it in the dark and trying to hide your body. A friend of mine's boyfriend couldn't believe the change in her after she'd been training for just a few weeks. She felt better about herself, so she was much more confident in bed.

If you're having sex and you look down at your belly and worry, that's not going to make you feel particularly sexy. It doesn't matter how big it is, but if it's toned, you'll be more likely to throw yourself into different positions.

An ex-girlfriend of mine was a former member of a girl band, but, when we first started seeing each other, she would turn the light out when we had sex and put the duvet on to walk to the bathroom. She would never let me see her walking around without her clothes on. Then she started exercising, and the next thing I knew she was in the kitchen cooking me breakfast naked. That all happened in the space of three months, and it was incredibly sexy to see her being so proud of her body.

Another of my clients is a multi-millionaire actor who I trained for the Emmys. His marriage wasn't in great shape, and he was on the verge of splitting up with his wife. He'd started to put on a bit of weight and, despite his wealth and fame, that made him lose confidence, and his sex life began to suffer more and more.

He also became increasingly needy, because he was feeling insecure, which was another big pressure on their relationship. He and his wife eventually went their separate ways, and he was devastated. However, we started training together and, within a couple of months, he was looking and feeling loads better. He got his confidence back, and he and his wife started seeing each other again. She fell in love with him all over again, because he was back to being himself, and they ended up getting back together.

I saw him shortly afterwards, and he thanked me for helping to get him and his wife reunited. He said he couldn't believe how much putting on weight had affected him mentally, and also his life as a whole. All it took was a few months to get things back on track, and now he's happier than ever.

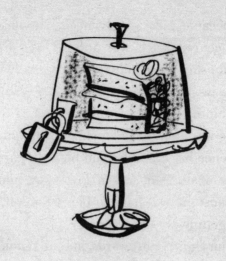

Chapter 3

The plan. If you're only going to read 18 pages, make it these

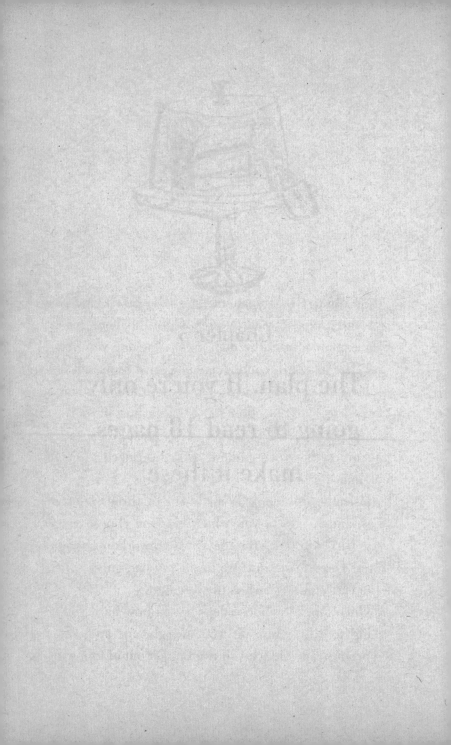

If you're a bit impatient (hey, who isn't?), and you only want to read one section of this book for an explanation of the plan, this is the one you need. The rest of the book has some great hints and tips for how to stay motivated, some inspirational success stories and loads of other helpful info but, if you just want to get started . . . ? Go for it. The next 18 pages are your quick reference guide to what you need to do to look amazing.

Basically, this book is made up of three different plans, and it's up to you which one you choose – the Lazy Girl workout, the Savvy Girl workout or the Fitness Queen workout. We think you can guess which is the easiest and which is the toughest.

Which one you choose depends on how hard you're willing to work, how fit you already are and, most importantly, how much you want to get out of following your chosen plan. Those on the Lazy Girl workout get to cheat occasionally and drink more alcohol than on the other two workouts, so it's all about being realistic about a) what you want to achieve and b) what you think you can stick to.

Also, the plans aren't set in stone. If you know you've got a week with a couple of parties coming up, you can switch down from the Fitness Queen or Savvy Girl workouts to the Lazy Girl for that week, if you fancy. And even though you may start out on the Lazy Girl workout, you can upgrade to Savvy Girl or Fitness Queen at any time. It's your choice.

The exercises

The Lazy Girl workout
This is for girls who haven't really exercised before and want to take it a bit more slowly.

In weeks 1 and 2, do two exercises from group A and one each from groups B and C

In weeks 3 and 4, do one exercise from groups A and C and two from group B

In weeks 5 and 6, do three exercises from group B and one from group C

The Savvy Girl workout
This is for girls who have exercised in the past and know they can get their fitness levels back up pretty quickly.

In weeks 1 and 2, do two exercises from group A, two from group B and one from group C

In weeks 3 and 4, do one exercise from group A, three from group B and one from group C

In weeks 5 and 6, do four exercises from group B and one from group C

The Fitness Queen workout
This is for girls who want to get the best results possible in the six weeks and are willing to work damn hard for it.

In weeks 1 and 2, do one exercise from group A, three from group B and one from group C

In weeks 3 and 4, do four exercises from group B and one from group C

In weeks 5 and 6, do five exercises from group B and one from group C

Group A
Each session should last 30–45 minutes

Netball
Rock climbing
Canoeing
Running
Rowing
Triathlon
Squash

Group B
Each session should last 45–60 minutes

Kettlebell training
Cycling
Hiking
Gymnastics
Tennis
Football
Swimming
Boxing
Gym session (including a variety of activities)

Group C
Each session should last 45–60 minutes

Salsa
Trampolining
Dancing
Swiss ball
Roller-skating
Aerobics class

The reason that we've given you such a broad range of exercises is because it's important to find some that suit you. No one sticks at anything they don't like for long, so it's really important to try things out and discover what you find fun to do. Loads of people go cycling because they enjoy it, not because it's some form of torture. Do you love rock climbing? Brilliant, do it twice a week. If you hate it when you try it? You never have to do it again. You can go rollerblading, play netball with friends or dance around your living room if that's what makes you happy and will keep you on track. What we're not saying is that you have to go running every day or spend all your time in the gym drinking protein shakes. Unless, of course, that's what you love doing. In which case, fabulous.

Let's face it, how many times have you spent half the night on the dance floor when you're out with your mates? That's still exercise, it's just that you're enjoying it, so you're not even noticing that you're moving your body around for hours on end and are probably getting quite tired. So the most important thing is to FIND EXERCISES YOU LIKE.

How can I find places to exercise in my area?

Your local-authority website will have a section where you can look up gyms near you. Also, if you have a local newspaper or magazine, it will have a section where people advertise things such as salsa classes, boxing clubs and climbing clubs. And you can even take a look on the noticeboard at your local supermarket for activities which you can take part in.

I'm quite lazy – can I still get fit?

Of course. You're only lazy when you're doing things you don't want to do. You're not lazy when there's a good party you want to go to, are you? No, because you want to be there. So, once you find the exercises you enjoy, you'll want to do them. And, once you start seeing results, you'll want to do them even more.

I'm lazy. Given the choice, I would lie in bed until midday every day, but I get up because I love what I do. When I run fitness boot camps – which I do several times a year – we're up at seven every morning, and I hate that part of it, but, as soon as we're exercising and everyone's enjoying themselves, I love it, and it all feels worthwhile.

On boot camp we do a series of different types of exercises – everything from canoeing to circuit training and swimming in the sea. Some people love the canoeing, some people hate it. Some people love the swimming, but one girl cried when she found out she had to do it. As the week goes on, people learn what they do and don't enjoy so, when they get back home, they can carry on with the things they do like. And they absolutely should not feel guilty about the things they don't like.

We all have different likes and dislikes, and you'll find your exercise loves through trial and error. And if you already know what they are? Fantastic, you won't have to waste any time trying things out.

I know from my years as a personal trainer that the time you stop enjoying the type of exercise you're doing is the time you give up, whether you're a lazy person or not. But, if exercise keeps you interested and doesn't seem like a chore, you'll be much more motivated. If I know that someone who is training with me loathes running, I'm not going to make them run every time they come and see me. What would be the point? They'll be running out the door before I know it.

The diet

On this plan, I want you to breakfast like a king, lunch like a prince and eat dinner like a pauper. What that basically means is that breakfast should be your main meal, lunch should be smaller and dinner smaller still. That way, your body has time to burn off your food during the day. It takes a while to get used to because we're conditioned to do it the other way round, but your body will soon adjust. The diet stays the same for the whole six weeks. There's no taking out or reintroducing foods, as I think that just gets confusing. You can use your wild card to enjoy something that's not on the plan but, if you're serious about losing weight and getting into shape, it shouldn't become a regular feature in your everyday diet.

Be prepared, though, as you may well experience some side effects in the early days of the diet. If you usually drink caffeine, you may find yourself sweating more and, if you're cutting out carbs and eating protein, you may get bad breath (so maybe warn friends and family!). Drinking lots of water will help to flush any toxins out of your body, and it's possible that you may get some spots as your body battles to get rid of all the nasty things that have been clogging up your insides. Don't worry, as all these things are only temporary and, in fact, they're a sign that your body is sorting itself out.

Here are some vital rules I'd like you to follow:

Eat after you train – never before

When you train, your body needs your blood to be going to your muscles and not to your digestive system, so it's best not to eat at all before you work out. If you wait until after you train, your metabolism will be high, and your blood will be pumping around more quickly than it would if you were resting. This means that all the good nutrients go to your muscles more quickly, and you burn the food off a lot faster, which means you gain less weight.

Protein of any kind is the best thing to eat after you've been training, because the protein will help repair the muscles. Eating vegetables will also help put good vitamins back in your body.

Eat when you're hungry

Whatever you do, don't skip meals. Think of your body as a fire that needs constant stoking. If you're hungry, eat. If you're going out and you know you're going to get hungry and want to nip into the nearest supermarket and grab a packet of crisps, be prepared. It's far better to snack on a piece of chicken or low-fat Greek yoghurt to keep you going between meals. Don't feel guilty about eating; this plan isn't about depriving yourself. If you do start missing meals, that's when you'll start feeling tired, hungry and demotivated.

Snack suggestions

Make sure your fridge is stocked with nice, healthy foods. Otherwise, you'll soon find yourself reaching for a bag of crisps, because they seem like the most convenient thing when you're hungry. Low-fat yoghurts, chicken, soups and crudités are all quick and easy things to nibble on and will help to stop you eating unhealthy snacks.

Cottage cheese
Low-fat Greek or natural yoghurt
Porridge
Crudités and salad
Soup (though avoid anything creamy)
Sugar-free muesli
Milk or soya milk
Berries
Eggs

Fish, chicken and lean meat

High in protein and lots of other essential nutrients but low in fat, these are great for getting into shape. Be careful how you prepare them though, if it's fried in loads of oil it'll do you no good. Grilling is always best.

Drinks

Drink two litres of water a day to help flush your system out. Water also helps with weight loss, because you can't break down fat if you're dehydrated. If you're exercising, you can drink up to four litres of water a day.

Fruit

Just have one piece of fruit a day, as it's very high in sugar. Fruits such as bananas, mangoes and strawberries are the worst culprits. Berries are the best fruit you can eat.

Herbs and spices

Use lots of herbs and spices, as they can really bring a dish to life. Add spices to stir fries instead of using thick sauces. Hot spices also help to stimulate your metabolism.

Vegetables

You can eat as many of these as you like, so try and make sure that vegetables play a really prominent part in your diet over the next six weeks.

Foods to avoid as much as possible:

Alcohol

If you're going to drink, vodka and slimline tonic and champagne are the best things to go for. But, no matter which way you look at it, unfortunately alcohol is never really going to do us any good. See page 87 for how alcohol fits in to the plan.

Fizzy drinks

Packed full of sugar, additives and caffeine. These are never going to be good for you, and don't be fooled by diet versions – they're just as bad.

Sauces

You can have ketchup occasionally, but avoid mayonnaise and other fatty sauces. Make some salsa, using tomatoes, herbs and chillis.

Caffeine

If you can, avoid all caffeine. It will take a few days to get out of your system, but you will feel so much better for it in the long term. Herbal teas such as green tea do contain some caffeine but, in the context of this plan, you can drink them. If you're missing a cup of tea in the morning, try hot water with a slice of lemon as an alternative.

Sugar

Ideally, you'll stay off all sugar on this plan, as it makes your blood-sugar levels rise quickly and then dip, leaving you feeling even hungrier and craving more sugar. Your body will soon get used to being without sugar but, if you are really craving it, you're far better off having some natural sugar such as berries rather than reaching for a bar of chocolate.

Nuts, seeds and avocados

I believe that fat is always fat, no matter what form it comes in, so, in the context of this plan, avoid high-fat foods such as nuts, seeds and avocados. Though the fat contained in these foods is completely different to what you'd see in a deep-fried Mars bar, and they do have a great many health benefits, this plan is primarily about losing weight, which is why we're reducing your fat intake. You will still be getting the fats you need from grilled meat, stir fries and other similar dishes.

I trained a lady a couple of years ago who was determined to lose weight. She was training five times a week with me and eating healthily, and she couldn't understand why she wasn't losing weight. I was also totally baffled, as she was working hard, so I told her to write down everything she was eating. She did and, when I saw her diet, it was perfect. I asked her if there was anything she had missed out, and she replied, 'Only the handful of nuts and seeds I have after every meal.'

She thought she was being healthy, but she was consuming so much extra fat and calories that all the exercise she was doing was being used to counteract all that new fat she'd built up rather than the existing weight she was looking to lose in the first place. It's no wonder she wasn't losing any weight. She cut out the nuts and seeds and, in a month, she'd lost a stone. I think that says it all.

Bread, pasta and potatoes

You don't actually need starchy carbs. Eating plenty of vegetables and meat will provide you with all the energy you need without making you put on weight. Carbs turn into sugar (or glucose) once you've taken them into your body. However if there is too much glucose in your body it ends up being stored as fat. So, if you don't exercise the carbs away, they become extra pounds. Research has shown that you carry starches such as beer, bread and pasta around the midriff area. Look at Italians – a lot of them have slim legs and big bellies, because they eat so much pizza and bread. If you are going to eat bread, remember that there are always healthier options you can go for. Basically, always go brown if you can. Most white bread you buy in shops is not only almost totally lacking in nutritional content, it's also packed with additives which will do you no good at all.

Cheese
Cheese is very high in fat. On the plus side, it does have calcium, but you can get that from milk.

Pesto
Pesto is shockingly high in fat. It's packed with Parmesan, pine nuts and olive oil, so just one jar can contain more than your entire daily recommended intake of fat.

Processed meat
Things such as salami may be delicious, but they're packed with fat to help the preservation process, so they're no good if you're trying to lose weight.

We're not stupid, and we know that there are times when it's going to be impossible to stick to the plan 100 per cent. And that's why we're giving you a bit of leeway – and a food wild card which you use once a week – because we're nice like that . . .

Here are the rules you need to stick to when following your chosen plan:

- Those following the Lazy Girl workout can drink

alcohol twice a week and use their food wild card once a week.

- Those following the Savvy Girl workout can drink alcohol once a week and use their food wild card once a week.

- The Fitness Queen can drink alcohol once a week, but she only has three food wild cards for the whole six weeks.

A word about cheating

Remember, a food wild card does not equal a massive blowout. And just because you have them, it doesn't mean you *have* to use them. They're to be reserved for an evening out, a special occasion or a nice treat. One wild card equals a nice sandwich or a baked potato, not a Thai takeaway with all the extras followed by a jumbo tub of ice cream.

The fact that you can drink once or twice a week isn't a licence to run to the pub after work. If you don't have to drink, don't drink. And you can't save all of your drinking nights up and go on a week-long binge either. If you want to win the body battle, you need to stick to the rules.

At the end of the day, if you overdo things, you're only cheating yourself, and you won't get the full results you want. And, remember, if you want to feel extra good about yourself, you can always up your exercise a notch the day after you've used your wild card.

Keeping a food diary

Many people like to keep food diaries but, although they can be really helpful, I certainly don't insist on them. We've included a template on our website (www.theredcarpetworkout.co.uk) It's surprising how much writing everything down wakes people up to those times when they don't even realize they're snacking.

Sample food plan

I've included the sample food plan over the page to give you an idea of what you should be eating, nothing here is set in stone, but hopefully this will help you when you come to plan your meals for the next six weeks.

THE RED CARPET WORKOUT

	BREAKFAST	SNACK	LUNCH	SNACK	DINNER
MON	Muesli with skimmed or semi-skimmed milk	Blueberries	Tuna salad (no mayo)	Low-fat Yoghurt	Grilled chicken with vegetables (no carrots or potatoes)
TUES	Porridge with berries	Low-fat yoghurt	Chicken salad (no mayo)	A couple of slices of peach	Grilled fish with vegetables
WED	Three egg-whites on wholemeal toast	Goji berries	Chicken & veg fajitas (no cheese or sour cream)	No snack	Steak with asparagus and mushrooms
THU	Muesli with skimmed or semi-skimmed milk	A pear	Leek & potato soup	Low-fat Yoghurt	Grilled fish with steamed greens (eg spinach)
FRI	Pepper, onion and mushroom omelette	Blueberries	Prawn salad (no mayo)	No snack	Chicken liver with green vegetables
SAT	Muesli with berries and skimmed or semi-skimmed milk	A handful of grapes	Chicken, tomato, cucumber and mint salad	An apple	Gazpacho followed by tuna tartare
SUN	Scrambled eggs with baked beans	Low-fat yoghurt	Roast (no potatoes or Yorkshire pudding!)	Low-fat sorbet	Tomato soup

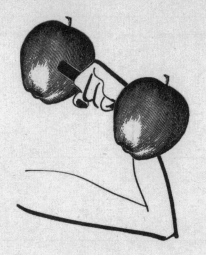

Chapter 4

What to expect, week by week

When will I start seeing results?

If you're being dedicated and you don't cheat, you should see results in a couple of weeks. But it's down to you how much effort you put in. You know what you need to do, but it's all about sticking to it and remembering that it *will* work.

If people think they can get away with eating rubbish and not exercising and still be slim, they will carry on eating rubbish and not exercising. But we all know that's not the reality. We'd all love to live on chocolate croissants and pizza (I know I would if I could) but, if you want to see results, you've got to stick to the plan and put in the time and effort. Just keep on reminding yourself that, after the six weeks, you're going to look amazing, and it will all be worth it.

What if I don't lose any weight in the first week? Or, even worse, what if I put some on?

Don't panic. Remember that this is a six-week plan, not a one-week plan. It's only natural that you're going to feel demotivated if you don't see results immediately, but you are guaranteed to see results in weeks two, three, and onwards from there, if you stick to the plan, and that will help to drive you on.

You will lose weight because the plan is built around science, not airy-fairy blue-sky thinking. You will experience body-changing weight loss, and your clothes will look better, because you're going to be more toned.

Eek! It's your first burst of exercise

Don't worry if you're out of breath and feel like giving it up and lying on the floor after two minutes when you first start to exercise. If you haven't worked out for a while, your body won't be used to it, but it's all about building up your resistance. And don't think you can't do it – if you think like that you'll have failed before you've even begun – just do what you can do and keep building it up and pushing yourself a little bit more time after time.

Set yourself little goals, and you'll feel amazing when you reach them. You wouldn't expect someone to come along and do your job with no training and help, so, by the same token, you're hardly likely to be able to run for miles on end straight away.

It's really important that you don't give yourself a hard time when you're starting out, as that makes you frustrated, which could cause you to give up. Everyone has to start somewhere – I've known some people who always considered themselves really lazy who have gone on to run marathons – so don't panic if you can't do a four-minute mile the first time you put your trainers on. Even a forty-minute mile is great, the fact that you've done it at all is great (what were you doing this time last week?), and you'll love that sense of achievement so much after you've done it that you'll probably want to give yourself a pat on the back!

The best advice when you're actually running is to concentrate on your breathing. Breathe in through your nose and out through your mouth and get into a rhythm. When I've trained boxers in the past, and they've been skipping, they always get into a rhythm, and that's how they can keep going for so long. It's all about finding your own pace. When you're concentrating on your breathing, it takes your mind off how far you've got left to run, and it keeps you feeling calm as well. Also, relax your shoulders. So many people tense up their shoulders, and that inhibits your running.

Week 1

In the first week, you will hate me slightly (don't worry, I can take it), and you'll probably (read: definitely) have some cravings. Sugar will be a big one, and also, if you're a big drinker, and you're going to places where you'd normally have wine with your dinner, then it's going to be hard. I know, I've been there and done it myself, and it hurt! You might feel tired and get a few niggles, but that's fine and to be expected, if you haven't done exercise in a while. If you get any soreness in your body, don't worry, it's just a build-up of lactic acid, and it won't take long to go away.

For the first three or four days, you'll be on a high and you'll feel really positive, and then you'll probably weigh yourself and you'll panic because you haven't lost weight instantly. Don't. Ideally, you should wait until the end of the second week to weigh yourself. But, if you simply have to weigh yourself, as long as you've been strict, you should expect to see a couple of pounds' weight loss. Don't expect the world, though; it's only the first week. And, if there isn't any weight loss in the first week, don't worry, because it will happen in the second week. Remember, people lose weight at different rates, so if your friend announces that she's dropped X amount of pounds, don't become despondent. The chances are, you'll lose more the following week.

I was training a female model recently who was trying to lose some of her post-pregnancy weight. Even though I asked her not to, she stepped on the scales at the end of week one and had only lost a pound. She felt really miserable, as if all her hard work had been for nothing. I told her to carry on training and not to panic – and also not to weigh herself again for at least another week. She did what I asked and, when she stepped on the scales again, she was four pounds lighter. Her hard work certainly felt worth it then.

I have one client who has been training with me for a while. She's just had her fiftieth birthday and was all excited because she'd been eating and drinking non-stop for ten days without doing any exercise and only put on a pound. She thought she'd got away with it but then, a week later, she weighed herself again and told me she'd put on five pounds in a day. Of course, she hadn't. The weight had built up during her binge, but it took a while to show on the scales. Some people will see weight gain and loss instantly while, for others, it takes a while to kick in, so don't panic if things don't change overnight.

Week 2

If you've enjoyed the first week, you'll enjoy the second week even more. And if you haven't enjoyed the first week, you will start to enjoy things in the second week, because your body is getting used to doing the exercise.

That said, you might find the diet part hard, and it's likely that your cravings will still creep in, because it does take a few weeks for your body to get used to its new eating pattern.

Weeks two and three are the times when you're most likely to fall off the wagon, because you're still near the beginning of the plan and may not feel totally dedicated to it yet. Stick with it, and you should lose another pound or two. You may not have lost anything in week one, but you may see a weight loss of three to four pounds in week two.

If your motivation is low, make sure you pamper yourself a bit and take time to relax when you're not working or exercising. And make sure you reward yourself when you do well – just not with chocolate or wine.

Week 3

Week three will be a transitional period, and you'll probably feel the least motivated of all the stages. But if you know that you'll probably feel a bit crappy, why not plan ahead and treat yourself to a nice massage, facial or a gorgeous new bag to help you deal with it?

You've had a couple of weeks of working hard, and I know that the thought of going for a run doesn't fill you with joy around now. But stick with it, because you're going to love me at the end of week six.

This is a turning point for you, and for many people week three is make or break. But remember that, when you get to the end of the week, you're halfway through.

You may not lose as much this week as you did in week two, which is another reason it may be hard not to throw your arms up in the air and dive into the nearest newsagent for stocks of chocolate, but you should definitely still see some movement on the scales.

Week 4

Week four is when you need to increase the intensity of your training. You also need to be strict with food, because you're over halfway through and you need to be more dedicated than ever. You need to step things up a level. Imagine the six weeks are gears on a car and, each week, you need to speed things up and work even harder.

You should see another pound or two of weight loss this week and, hopefully, that will spur you on to work even harder in the final two weeks. You're so close now to the end that not putting in the maximum effort would make no sense. When that energy boost kicks in, you feel so good that it becomes addictive, which should spur you into staying on track.

You should also start to see really good changes in your body this week. Your muscle tone will have improved, you'll find exercise easier and you should have tons more energy. Your clothes should also feel different on you, and those niggling bits of excess fat you've been desperate to get rid of should be getting smaller by the day.

Week 5

You're on the home stretch, so you should be feeling really good about things. You should see even more changes in your body, and around a two- to three-pound weight loss. If you've been putting off trying on your skinny jeans while you've been on the programme, now is the time to do it. You'll be surprised how different they look and feel, and that should give you a massive boost.

Any particular parts of your body that you've specifically targeted will experience a real change. If you've been trying to tone your arms, do the bingo-wings wobble test and see how much less they shake about. If you've been working your abs hard, you should be able to wear a tight-fitting top without giving it a second thought.

Give yourself a massive pat on the back with every little bit of change you notice, because it will be those things that make you want to work harder than ever.

You'll be looking great in week five, and just think how fabulous you're going to look at the end of next week.

Week 6

This is the week when I usually take my clients and work them into the ground. You need to up your exercise by a couple of sessions and be as strict as you possibly can be on the food front, remembering not to skip meals. Just eat lots of lean protein and vitamin-packed vegetables, and drink a lot of fluids and good-quality green tea.

Don't be surprised to see a loss of about three to five pounds at the end of the week. But it isn't just about how much weight you've lost on the scales, it's about how you look in a certain dress or pair of jeans you've been dreaming about wearing. And if you've stuck to the plan, you're going to look bloody fantastic.

If you want to up the ante in the final week...

That special event is about to roll around, and you want to look your absolute best. If you want to *really* speed things up in the last week of the plan, it's pretty straightforward – you have to be super strict and cut your calories down and increase your exercise a lot.

I would never ask you to do something like this at the beginning of the programme, because it's too big a step but, by this point, you should feel pretty motivated, and you will also have it in mind that you're nearing the end and the strictness will only last a matter of days.

Try and exercise for around an hour every day and have something very light to eat before you go to bed, such as tomato soup.

Remember: you don't have to follow this section of the plan if you don't want to. This is just another option for those who want to go for the burn in the last week.

It's the day of a party, how do I get a flat stomach?

Avoid all fizzy drinks, even carbonated water, as they create bloating. Also avoid chewing gum, as this has the same effect. And don't eat and drink at the same time. You shouldn't drink when you eat in any case, as it confuses the digestion process. Ideally, you should drink forty minutes after eating, to rehydrate.

Starchy carbs such as pasta and potatoes make you bloated because you carry them around your midriff, so avoid them as well.

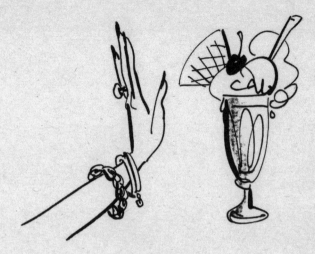

Chapter 5

Drinking and the fun stuff. Oh, and how to stop making excuses . . .

How often can I drink?

A lot of people think you can't drink and get fit, but you can if you're clever about it. In the context of the plan, try to stick to just one night's drinking per week (two if you're a Lazy Girl). The best things to drink are either champagne, or vodka or gin with slimline tonic or soda and fresh lime. These are what I'd call 'clean' drinks, because they don't have many additives. Laurent Perrier Ultra Brut is the least calorific champagne. It was the only champagne Kate Moss had at her last birthday party, which says a lot.

Drinks such as cider and lager are the worst things to have because they bloat you out and make you feel uncomfortable, and who wants to spend all night feeling as if their dress no longer fits them properly? They also contain the highest number of calories – you might not think it, but a pint of lager is absolutely packed with sugar.

The problem with alcohol is often not the drinks themselves, it's how they make you feel the following day. You're tired, you'll have food cravings and you'll want sugar and salt so much you wouldn't believe it. Worse still, your willpower will be at an all-time low, and that's when the lardy yellow foods start to creep in. And one binge can lead to a downward spiral because booze often gives people what I like to call the 'beer fear': they get themselves in such a state because they've cheated that they can't see it as a one-off and a bit of a blip but instead as the beginning of the end of healthy eating.

If you want some kind of motivation to stop you drinking more than once a week, when you get home after a night of non-drinking, put the money you would have spent on alcohol to one side and, at the end of the six weeks, count it up and go shopping. You'll be shocked at how much you've saved

Stop making eating excuses

It's too easy to make excuses to explain why you can't follow a healthy eating plan. There are ways around every situation and, nine times out of ten, you can avoid having to eat foods which you know aren't good for you. No one is going to lose weight for you. And, no matter how convincing your excuses, the only person you're going to fool is yourself. It's up to you to choose the best option in every situation.

You have to exercise some restraint, because there are always going to be temptations. Okay, imagine you're out to dinner with your boyfriend. You really like him but, when he pops to the toilet, a really hot guy who you know is a player walks in and asks you out. Do you a) Give him your number and come clean with your boyfriend? b) Give him your number and lie to your boyfriend about it? or c) Tell him you're not interested?

If you give him your number and lie to your boyfriend, you're really only cheating yourself, because you're putting everything at risk and you could lose the guy you like for a flash in the pan. It's the same with food – if you eat things you shouldn't, the only person you're hurting is yourself. And if you're in denial about the fact that you're eating bad things, you're only cheating yourself and putting your weight loss at risk.

If you keep making the same mistakes over and over again, nothing is going to change with you internally or externally.

It's the same as if you keep giving a hot playboy your

number every time you're with a nice guy – you're going to end up lonely, because you're not learning your lessons. And while the playboy may be exciting for that moment, you'll be left feeling guilty and upset with yourself.

How to cope in tempting situations

They're always going to be there, but there are ways to behave yourself when temptation comes knocking – even if it does look like a delicious jam doughnut. If you're prepared for these situations, then half the battle is already won.

Plan your bad days in advance, because there's no use pretending that you're not going to have them. If you have a work event or someone's birthday do or wedding coming up, the chances are that you're going to want to drink alcohol. It's also unlikely that you'll have a choice when it comes to what you eat, and taking your own plastic container full of chicken salad to a wedding looks a bit odd.

If you know that these parties are coming up, you can plan around them and try and squeeze in an extra exercise session or eat even more healthily than usual the day before.

Basically, we're saying that, if you want to go out and

enjoy yourself, do. Just don't let one night out mean that you totally fall off the wagon and spend all of the next day munching on biscuits and fast food.

As long as you know you have those days scheduled in, you can plan around them so you won't feel too guilty the next day. So, when you're planning your nights out, also plan how you're going to counteract their effects.

Holidays in the Sun

The problem with holidays in the sun is that everyone likes to drink a lot. And when you drink a lot, the following day, you crave things that are bad for you, such as cheese, bread, fizzy drinks and fried food. As soon as you wake up after a night out, they're the things you're going to want to eat, and they're the worst things you can fill your stomach with.

The best way to get rid of your cravings is to go for a jog. I know that sounds crazy and extreme, and you can't imagine yourself ever doing it, but it works. It's what I do if I've got a hangover since, otherwise, I know I'd want to have a ridiculously greasy breakfast and then end up writing off the day, probably eating more rubbish because I've had a bad start.

Going for a jog will go against everything you want to do, but you'll thank yourself for it. If you really can't face the thought of exercise on the morning after far too many cocktails, minimize the damage. Instead of reaching for the nearest croissant, have a healthy breakfast which will help balance your blood-sugar levels. An unbuttered piece of toast – bread isn't recommended, generally, in the plan but, if it's going to stop you going off the rails completely, it's fine in this instance – with two poached eggs on top is a million times better than having sugary things.

If you want something with it, have some baked beans and some grilled mushrooms and tomatoes. That's like a healthy fry-up, without any of the frying, obviously. Stay away from sausages and bacon because they're high in fat, but if you want something extra, have some salmon.

Swimming is also great when you're feeling hungover and, if you're on a beach holiday, it should be really convenient, but you do need to exert yourself. If you like the idea of going for a power walk, avoid doing it on the beach. Sand is an uneven surface, so you really up your chances of injuring yourself. So many of my clients have hurt themselves walking or running on sand, so stick to flat surfaces.

Mediterranean breaks
Things such as olives, quiche and cheese are terrible for you if you're trying to lose weight, but they are very popular in Mediterranean countries. A lot has been

made recently of the beneficial effect all the olive oil in the Mediterranean diet has on things such as heart disease and longevity and, though there's a great deal of truth in this, it's also true that olive oil is very high in fat, so it's still going to stop you shedding those pounds. In the Med it's also the norm to drink wine during the day, but don't get into a routine of doing this, because it's a hard habit to break.

However, the fabulous thing about places such as Italy, Greece and France is that they're really into their fresh, seasonal vegetables (which always seem to taste so much nicer there than they do in Britain), and they also have a lot of grilled fish, steak and lean chicken on the menu, so it won't be hard to follow the plan. There's nothing to stop you going for a run or a hike either, a fantastic opportunity to see the local area and take in a bit of picturesque scenery as you get fit!

Skiing holidays
It's easy to fall into the trap of thinking you're doing exercise and burning off calories when you're skiing, but the way I see it, you're only sliding down a hill, so that doesn't mean you can go off and indulge afterwards.

Obviously, because it's cold, you want to eat more, and the après ski means that you drink hot things such as hot chocolate and Baileys. In the past, I've always put on the most weight of any holiday when I go skiing, because all I want to do is eat comfort food and drink brandy. I have to really watch myself.

As a general rule, when you're on holiday, if you're tempted to eat unhealthily, don't drink as well.

Going down the pub

As I've already explained earlier in the book, the best things you can drink are either vodka and slimline tonic or champagne. If your budget doesn't stretch to champagne, you can have sparkling wine, although it does have more additives in it, so it's not as 'clean' as champagne, and it's also sweeter, which can make you feel hungrier.

If you're eating, have a steak or some grilled chicken or fish with lots of vegetables. And have rice instead of a baked potato or chips. Lots of pubs also do salmon fillets now, so that's a good option.

Try not to dig your hands into other people's fatty snacks, such as crisps and nuts. It's surprising how quickly the calories rack up when you're grazing.

If everyone's heading off to the kebab shop after the pub and you're too hungry to say no, the best thing to have is a chicken shish kebab with salad. But hold off on the sauces, because that's where you'll slip up.

Cinema

If you can't help but snack at the cinema, go for some salted popcorn, which is the best of a bad bunch. But check with the kiosk, because sometimes they add extra butter to it so, needless to say, it instantly becomes a *very* unhealthy snack. Stay away from pretty much everything else, especially fizzy drinks, sweet popcorn and hot dogs.

Bowling

Food at bowling lanes tends to be very fatty and fast-food based. A lot of places will do a chicken-fillet burger, so you're best off having one of those, without mayonnaise. Have some salad and a bit of ketchup. And, if you can bear it, don't have the bun.

The late-night munchies

You normally get hungry late at night because you're thirsty, so have some water. If you're sure you are hungry, have some cottage cheese or a low-fat yoghurt, because they'll fill you up.

The mid-morning slump

This is when most people reach for a bar of chocolate because they've had a sugary breakfast and it's caused their blood-sugar levels to rise and then fall sharply again. If you've had a balanced breakfast with protein, you shouldn't experience this but, if you are craving sugar, the best thing you can do is have some fruit. Berries are great for filling you up, and they have really good antioxidant properties.

It's always hard to avoid the office sweets, and that's where a lot of people put on weight. If you don't think you can keep your hands off the biscuits and sweets that are lying around, fill in the food diary from the website on a daily basis. By writing everything down, you'll realize how much you're snacking – sometimes when you're not even really hungry. Again, this is one of those situations where, if you've already prepared and got some healthy snacks ready in your drawer, then you'll be better placed to fight temptation.

Party canapés

Sadly, most party canapés are loaded with fat and calories. The worst ones are mini-burgers. Anything with pastry is bad and, obviously, anything battered should be totally avoided. Sushi is great, and chicken satay without the fatty satay sauce is also fine.

A good tip is to eat dinner before you go to a party so that you're not tempted by all the trays that are heading past If you don't have time to eat, try not to drink alcohol until after you've had your fill of canapés. As soon as you have a drink or two, your resolve goes, and you'll be throwing down the mini-quiches before you realize what you're doing.

PMT

All women get those hormonal urges, so it's always good to prepare for them. If you know they're coming, have some snacks on hand to satisfy your cravings. If you want to have a piece of chocolate, it's not the end of the world. But don't keep a huge bar on your desk, just keep a little. Otherwise, you may well find yourself mindlessly eating whatever's there. That said, you should find that the exercise you're doing will help fight the effects of PMT.

Tiredness

Berries are great for giving you an energy kick, and they'll keep your energy levels much more stable than, say, a sugary cup of tea or some biscuits. These will only give you a temporary boost and will ultimately leave you feeling even more tired.

Christmas

The most important thing at Christmas is not to start digging into all the nibbles. Most of them may look fairly harmless, because they're small, but they're loaded with fat and calories. If you want to snack, have things such Parma ham, chicken skewers or sushi.

When it comes to alcohol, if you drink beer all day, you're swallowing down loads of calories and you'll feel very bloated. Stick to wine or champagne, and drink loads of water in between, which will help to make you feel fuller too and will lessen the desire to snack.

When it comes to the big Christmas dinner, have lots of meat and vegetables and just one or two potatoes and a bit of stuffing, and avoid Yorkshire puddings, as they're often cooked in lots of oil. Stay away from the really sweet stuff too. Have Christmas pudding, but no brandy butter, for instance.

Most importantly, remember that Christmas is only one day (no matter what the shops might tell you), so don't take it as an excuse to eat bad foods and drink booze for weeks on end. And there's nothing wrong with going for a jog on Boxing Day, is there? If you get an iPod for Christmas, strap it on and go for a run.

If you suffer from SAD

I know that in those dreary weeks after Christmas, the only thing you really want to do is hide under your duvet, eat comforting food and watch bad television. You feel exhausted and irritable for no real reason you can think of, and your motivation is lower than at any other time of the year. But for many people, when the nights draw in is actually when they feel most rewarded by the programme, because exercise is the best thing possible to help counteract them feeling tired and sluggish. Not only will exercise get you out and about in the fresh air and light, but like I've said earlier, exercise in general really helps to lift your mood.

The winter months are generally when everyone is feeling most short of money, too, as a result of Christmas spending, so it's a great time to make use of your gym membership and make sure that it doesn't go to waste. Go the gym instead of going out and you'll save yourself a fortune.

Easter
When it comes to chocolate, choose your favourite egg and give the rest away. Really enjoy it, and don't give yourself a hard time about it, and don't think that, just because you've had one, you have to have five.

Remember: like Christmas, Easter is only one day.

Summer nights
There's always a temptation to sit outside on summer nights drinking rosé and snacking on unhealthy foods, so I always recommend that, if you are going to do that, have a proper meal first, so you're not tempted by crisps and nuts. Being full also means that you're likely to drink less.

Summer is also when everyone has barbecues, so it's easy to stick to the plan, because there's always plenty of meat and salads available. Barbecues don't need to just be about sitting around eating burgers, they're a great time for trying out new salads as well as getting stuck in to delicious grilled fish and vegetables. Have a piece of chicken and salad instead of a hot dog and coleslaw, and you can stick to the plan, no problem. It's about making the right choices.

Birthdays or a romantic meal

No one can be good all the time. If you've got a special occasion coming up and you want to indulge, do it! Just don't then see it as the first step to going back to unhealthy eating and giving up on everything. See it as a one-off, enjoy it and then do some exercise and eat healthily for the following few days.

I don't sit around on Christmas Day or my birthday nibbling raw broccoli and drinking hot water and lemon, I have wine and I have a nice meal. But I don't then carry on the celebrations for several more days. I spoil myself, and I move on, and you should do the same.

Don't panic if you slip up.

We've budgeted for a bit of failure. As I've said before, this is a six-week plan not a ten-minute crash diet. We could easily have put together a 'lose seven pounds in seven days' plan, but that's not realistic. It's not healthy, it's not sustainable, and the weight will pile back on as soon as you stop following it to the letter.

The idea of the Red Carpet Workout is to give you a

decent amount of time to really change the way you think about food and exercise so, hopefully, you're not going to see it as a fad. There are some great health and fitness lessons that you can learn and use effortlessly in your everyday life, even after you've come to the end of the six weeks. This is a balanced, all-round plan that will work on getting your body in shape long-term; it's not just about dropping a few pounds on the scales (although that is nice too).

Because you've got forty-two days of the Red Carpet Workout, if you do have one day where you're a bit badly behaved, it doesn't mean that the other forty-one don't count. Whereas, if you're doing a seven-day plan and you have a day of overindulgence, the chances are you're going to abandon the whole thing. We all have days when we're stressed or when something upsets us and, before we know it, we've stuffed ourselves with comfort foods. But, if you do have a bad day, remember that, in the grand scheme of things, it's not a massive problem. Just get back to being good the next day.

Whatever you do, if you falter, just get back on the plan and *do not give yourself a hard time*. This is totally counter-productive and will make you feel weak. Why not just promise yourself you'll add another day on to the end of your six weeks instead? That makes a lot more sense than wasting all the good work you've already done.

As soon as you have a blip, take a step back and look at everything you've achieved in the days before and at how proud you feel, and also think of what you can achieve afterwards. That should spur you on to start afresh. Take a minute to remember why you're following this plan in the first place (if you filled it in, have a look at the goal chart). The thought of how much better you'll look and feel after having completed the programme is often enough motivation in itself.

That's why I let you drink – I'm a realist. I know you're probably going to do it anyway, so I'd rather manage your expectations so that you won't be berating yourself if you party for a night or two a week. I'm letting you make mistakes. I'm not expecting you to fail, because you won't, but we're only human, and no one's perfect, so there is a buffer zone if you misbehave.

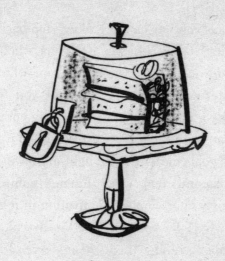

Chapter 6

From Pret to Pizza Express . . . The essential eating-out guide

There are going to be times – whether it's a work do or just meeting up with a friend – when you're going to find yourself out for lunch or dinner and tempted by the delicious menu. But a nice meal doesn't mean that you have to fall spectacularly off the wagon.

That's why we've created this eating-out guide – so you can make sensible choices and have a great time without feeling regretful afterwards. Think of this guide in terms of the 'best of a bad bunch'. If you do have to eat at the following restaurants, or at takeaways and other food outlets these are the best choices you can make.

As you'll have seen from the diet-plan section of the book, bread is a no-no, so if you are going to eat a sandwich, you have to use your wild card. And, as a general rule, when it comes to sandwiches, avoid anything with full-fat mayo, even if it's masquerading as a healthy choice.

It's easy to be tempted by all the other tasty things that are on offer when you walk into a restaurant or coffee shop but, remember, you can have that creamy sauce or a brownie in six weeks – so stay strong for now! And, weirdly, at the end of the six weeks, you may find that you don't actually want it any more . . .

This guide is also brilliant for after-plan maintenance and shows that you can carry on eating well, wherever you go, just by making the right choices.

Strada

Starters
Bresaola

Gamberoni

Zuppa di pasta e fagioli

Mains
Insalata Nizzarda

Salmone con lenticchie

Bistecca di manzo

Spigola al forno

Pizza Express

Starters
Insalata del sole

Mains
Nostrana salad
Pollo verdure salad

Café Rouge

Starters
French onion soup (without Gruyère cheese)
Mussels

Mains
Salade de la mer
Salmon à la Niçoise
Demi poulet

TGI's

Starters
Wicked Chicken
(this is not recommended, it's a last resort!)

Mains
Fillet steak (no sauce)
Wicked Chicken
Jack Daniel's® salmon
BBQ chicken salad
All with vegetables or salad

Zizzi

Pollo or Niçoise salad (Everything else is bad)

Wagamama

Starters
Grilled chicken gyoza

Mains
Chilli chicken or seafood ramen

Drinks
Raw juice or fruit juice

Nando's

Mains
All grilled chicken
Rice as side (if you're having this at lunch,
otherwise you'll need to use your wild card)
Corn on the cob
Mediterranean chicken salad

Curry houses

Starters
Lamb chops
Chicken and prawn tikka

Mains
Mixed grill with side salad

Avoid anything with sauce, as it usually has ghee in it,
which is clarified butter. As always, stay away from
bread, potatoes and rice.

Chinese restaurants

Starters
Won ton soup
Chicken satay (no sauce)

Mains
Prawns or chicken with mushrooms
Crispy duck

Chinese is mainly all bad so, really, you want to stay away from anything fried and all noodles. Most sauces are terrible if you're looking to lose weight, so the drier the dish the better. No rice!

Thai restaurants

Starters
Thai beef or prawn salad
Chicken satay with no sauce

Mains
Pad rad prik or similar steamed-fish dishes

Stay away from the pad Thai, all sauces and, specifically, curries.

Japanese restaurants

Starters
Edamame beans
Miso soup

Mains
Any kind of sashimi
Salads
Miso cod
Wagyu or kobe beef

Greek restaurants

Starters
Fava beans
Tzatziki
Greek salad (no feta or bread)

Mains
Pork souvlaki
Kleftiko (no potatoes)
Any grilled fish

British/Mediterranean restaurants

Starters
Any soup that doesn't have cream
Gazpacho
Tuna or salmon tartare
Grilled prawns
Grilled chicken or meat skewers
Mixed grilled veg

Mains
Tuna steak
Chicken dishes (without cheese or creamy sauces)
Steaks
Grilled fish (no sauce)
Lamb shank

Sides
Beans and pulses
Vegetables

Obviously, you need to avoid all desserts and stay away from too many fruit juices and too much alcohol. Stick to water, and you'll save a fortune on your bill!

There's also the everyday dilemma of lunch time. Maybe your choices of places to grab something to eat are limited, or you're rushing out to meet friends and you don't want to find yourself tempted by fatty bar foods. So what are the best choices you can make in fastfood restaurants and sandwich shops?

Remember that it's very easy to slip back into those old habits and pick up crisps and chocolate to munch with your sandwich, especially when they come as part of a good-value meal deal. Half the time you do it without even thinking, and yet you probably don't either want or need them. Have your sandwich, and then wait for a while. If you still feel hungry, have a piece of fruit or another of the healthy snacks already listed in the book to fill you up. Having said all this, if you really want to control what you're eating, the best thing you can possibly do is make your lunch at home.

Subway

Subway club
Sweet onion chicken terayaki
Ham and chicken breast
(These all have under 6g of fat)

Stay away from the crisps and fizzy drinks here, and don't be lured into buying the meal deal, even if it might save you fifty pence.

Starbucks

Roast British chicken breast and roasted tomato
sandwich (this has under 5 per cent fat)
Tuna mayo sandwich (this has under 5 per cent fat)
Roasted chicken salad with mange touts wrap
(this has under 3 per cent fat)
Mild chilli chicken malted wheat panini
(but avoid all other paninis)
Fruit salad

Say no to all desserts – even skinny muffins – and if you
must have a coffee, have a Frappaccino Light with
sugar-free hazelnut syrup

Costa Coffee

Free-range egg sandwich
Roast chicken sandwich
Tuna salad sandwich
Arrabiata chicken panini
Cajun chicken flatbread

If you must have coffee, a cappuccino is best or, better
still, have a healthy green tea.

JOE FOURNIER

Upper Crust

Ham salad
Chicken salad

These should only be eaten as a last resort.

Boots

Carrot sticks
Fruit salad
All Shapers salads
Sushi selection
All Shapers sandwiches and wraps

Eat

Chicken salad sandwich
Crayfish and lime sandwich
Smoked beef and horseradish sandwich
Tuna and red-onion sandwich
Turkey and cranberry sandwich
All soups except anything with cream
Spicy crayfish salad
Bean salad

115

THE RED CARPET WORKOUT

Breakfast bacon butty
Yoghurt, muesli and mixed berries
Porridge
Swiss Bircher muesli

Pret a Manger

All of the 'Slim' range of sandwiches are good,
except for the All-day Breakfast
Bean and herb soup
Lentil turmeric soup
Miso soup (great)
Salmon crayfish salad (amazing)
Deluxe sushi

Drinks
Water
Carrot juice
Vitamin Volcano
Pomegranate Power

Marks and Spencer

Grilled chicken breast pieces
(chicken tikka pieces are good)

Ham and egg roll
Low-fat tuna and sweetcorn sandwich
Low-fat chicken sandwich with mayo
Tuna salad
Salmon salad
Carrot and celery sticks

McDonald's, KFC, Burger King

What are you doing even walking into one of these places? If you ever find yourself in a place that has photos of burgers on the wall, turn around and walk out immediately.

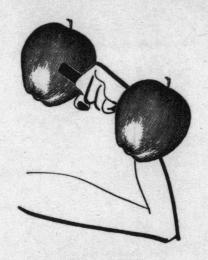

Chapter 7

Everything you need to know about exercise – and some fascinating facts

The do's and don'ts of exercise

- Starting a new exercise regime is all about making sure you're prepared. This doesn't mean going out and spending a fortune on all the latest fitness gear – you can work out in a ten-year-old T-shirt and some pyjama bottoms if that's what you feel comfortable in. But always make sure you have a decent pair of trainers. It's no good running in a pair of £2.99 pumps, because you could end up injuring your body. Ideally, if you can afford it, go somewhere that specializes in running shoes, get measured properly and buy the shoes that are right for you.

- Unless you know that you're 100 per cent sure you're going to use it, don't buy an exercise bike or treadmill for home. They generally end up as a clothes horse or something that gets moved to your shed before being put on eBay. You're better off saving your money and joining a gym or tennis club instead. Remember, you must do something you enjoy, or it won't last.

• You start burning calories as soon as you start exercising, but you only start burning fat after twenty minutes, so your workouts should always last thirty minutes or more.

• Avoid quick fixes, such as vibrating machines. These things are marketed really well, and they are made to seem as if they are the easy way out. I'm all about making exercise as easy as possible so, if I thought they worked, I would buy twenty and make all my clients use them. But they're not what they seem. They work for a small amount of time, and then your body gets used to the movement and they don't do anything more.

• Don't over-train. If you're really sore in one area but think you can work through it, you may injure yourself. If you're feeling sore in a certain place, exercise a different part next time. Don't put too much pressure on your body.

- Don't overdo it. If the weight is too heavy for you to lift, or the run is too far for you, don't do it. Yes, you do need to push yourself, but you don't want to put yourself off these things for life or, even worse, hurt yourself. Equally, don't do things that you find too easy, because you'll get bored very quickly.

- If you're trying something you've never done before, make sure you get correct supervision. For instance, don't try and go rock climbing without getting some form of training.

- Don't listen to friends who think they know more than you do. That's the biggest cause of injury. Just because someone's been going to a gym for a few months, it doesn't mean that they're knowledgeable. If in doubt, ask a professional. I remember, years ago, I was in the gym, and my friend's dad was there. He was a body-builder so, when he told me how I should be doing things, I believed him. I ended up with a bad neck for months as a result.

- Do find stuff you enjoy. I know I keep repeating this, but that's because it is *so* important. If you don't enjoy exercise, you won't want to do it. Full stop.

- Find something you know you can stick to. Don't take up salsa somewhere that's thirty miles away, because the chances are you'll give up after the first class. Exercise needs to be accessible.

- Always mix exercises up. Your body gets used to doing the same thing and doesn't work as hard, so it's good to keep your exercise routine varied so it works harder. If you were to drink the same amount of alcohol every day for a year, eventually you would stop getting drunk, because your body would become immune to it. And it's the same with exercise – if you follow the same pattern over and over again, your body will get used to it. When I train people, we never do the same thing twice in a short space of time. This makes the body more efficient, and you burn more calories. I'd recommend starting your workout with a bit of cardio activity (like a run or a cycle ride) and follow it with three or four of the exercises below, such as sit-ups or press-ups. You shouldn't do these more than twenty times each.

- Always wind down properly after exercising. It's important to wind down after exercise (see page 142 for an explanation as to why). Keep moving, but move slowly. If you're running, run more slowly, or walk. If you're swimming, just step the pace down a bit. And, if you're lifting weights, make sure you stretch before you finish. Reduce the intensity of what you're doing to get the oxygen back in your body, which will get rid of the lactic acid. Don't just lie on the floor and give up! You need to warm down slowly.

What benefits does each kind of exercise have for me?

Running

Running burns lots of calories, and it's really good for your legs and your stomach – in particular your obliques – because of the rotation movements you make when you're running. That's why sprinters always have great six-packs.

Walking

Walking is very low impact and is something which is good to start off with, but you need to challenge yourself. Walk uphill if you can, because that will burn more calories, and it will also help to tone your legs and bum.

Boxing

Boxing is cardiovascular and burns fat, and it's all about the rotation and twisting movements, as well as using your legs. It's also great for stress relief. You can do it either with gloves against a punchbag or a friend wearing pads, or you can box into air like a shadow boxer, so you won't even need an opponent!

There are six basic moves with boxing, and they take a matter of minutes to learn. I've discovered from my years of training people that, while a lot of women are quite anti-boxing at first, they soon grow to love it. It doesn't have to be some macho contest to break the other person's nose; in fact, it's great fun to do with a friend. Once you've bought the equipment, it will last you for years.

These are the six basic moves you need to know:

1. The jab

This is a straight arm punch with your leading arm – whether you're right- or left-handed. You stand slightly side-on with your front foot pointed towards one o'clock and your back foot pointing towards three o'clock. Bend at the knees and have your shoulders slightly forward in an aggressive position, then shift your weight from your back leg to your front leg and jab your arm. Extend the arm and bring it back; don't just leave it there. Ultimately, you want to connect using the two big first knuckles on your hand, because they're the ones that are connected to bone. The others aren't, so you'll bruise your hand if you hit with the two side knuckles. Don't tuck your thumb inside the fist, tuck it into the side.

2. The cross
This is a punch across the body where you rotate and twist the hips and punch forward. Use the same stance as before, put your weight on the front leg, and use the opposite arm to punch through, using your hips to rotate as fast as you can to provide the power. Imagine that your wrist is a loaded spring and punch out and then bring it back. Again, just use the first two knuckles to hit with.

3. The left hook
Use the same stance, rotate towards your front right leg and come through with a punch with the opposite arm cocked in a hooking movement. Rotate as fast as you can using your legs to power the punch, not just your arms.

4. The right hook
This is exactly the same move as the left hook, above, but on the opposite side.

5. The upper cut
Using the same stance, dip the hips slightly and punch upwards, putting all your weight on your front leg as you do so. You want to hit towards the ceiling, imagining you're hitting someone under the chin.

6. Upper cut 2
This is exactly the same move, on the opposite side.

Now you know the moves, you can do combinations of them, in whatever way you feel comfortable with.

Swimming
Swimming has always been known as a great, all-round exercise, but lots of people don't get the most of it because they don't push themselves. It's enjoyable, and they stay at a slow, steady rate, so they may as well be going on a slow walk. It's much better to do two lengths as fast as you can, have a minute's rest and then go again rather than do ten laps slowly, which won't really get your heart rate going.

Tennis and squash

Tennis and squash are both great, as you play against a friend or partner, which often motivates you to be more competitive and push yourself. They get your heart rate up, because you run around a lot, and this burns lots of calories. Squash is very explosive and helps you gain lean muscle mass. Only play squash if you don't have any form of heart disease, or leg and ankle problems, because it is very high impact. Tennis is similar to squash. It's not as intense, but it's great for your abdominals, because of the turning movements. It's also great for your arms – look at Rafael Nadal.

Yoga and Pilates

I've always gone a bit against accepted wisdom when it comes to yoga, in that I'm not a big fan of its exercise benefits. It's great for body tone, and most of my clients do it and love it, but, in the context of this plan, it doesn't count as one of your exercises. Do it by all means, if you enjoy it, but you need to see it as an added extra.

Pilates is great if you're using bands, because it really makes you work, and it's like doing resistance training, but, if I use it in training, I mix it in with other, higher-impact exercises.

Basically, Pilates and yoga will help to tone you up, but, if you're looking to burn calories, it's not going to do that as well as the cardiovascular exercises I've listed above. I'd recommend it as being better for part of your maintenance after you've completed the plan rather than as an aid to losing weight quickly.

Netball

Netball is brilliant cardiovascular exercise. It's fabulous for your legs, and you're rotating a lot, so it's good for your stomach. What's more, it's a fun activity, so it helps to take your mind off the fact that you're exercising. I find that, for lots of the people I train, playing netball is an excuse to take up something they used to love at school but, for one reason or another, haven't done in years.

Football

Football is another really good cardiovascular exercise, and it's a fantastic sport to take up if you're not hugely slim, since a bit of body fat will enable you to work hard for the ninety minutes of the game.

Rock climbing

Rock climbing is excellent for working the muscles in your upper back and in your legs. It's also brilliant for abdominals, because you need to keep your core nice and tight when you're doing it.

Rowing and canoeing

Canoeing and rowing are fabulous for your abdominal areas – your obliques and intercostals. It's also great for back and shoulder muscles, and very cardiovascular.

Cycling

Cycling is a low-impact exercise, but it's something you can do for a long time, perhaps combined with a twenty-minute run afterwards.

Salsa dancing

Salsa gets your legs, hips and bum moving. It's not amazing for weight loss but it's great for toning.

Trampolining

Trampolining is superb exercise but, despite what people think, it's very technical, so you do need a coach. It's cardiovascular and lots of fun.

Gymnastics

There are plenty of gymnastics centres throughout the UK where you can go as an adult, pay a fee and take a class. It's not only cardiovascular but it's brilliant for toning.

Rollerskating

This is very low intensity – but it's better than doing nothing.

Dancing

Dancing on a night out is fabulous, as long as there's water or champagne in your glass rather than a creamy cocktail.

Kettlebell training

You need to get someone to show you how to train with this initially but, once you've mastered it, it's fantastic for toning, and especially for working your core muscles and your legs. It's very explosive and helps with weight loss, as it burns a lot of calories.

Swiss balls

Swiss balls are excellent aids, fabulous for spot-toning loads of different areas, but you need to do some cardiovascular exercise as well.

Hiking

Hiking is fantastic, but you need to work at speed. It's far better to do a half-hour hike at a decent speed than a two-hour hike at a slow speed.

What are the best exercises for the specific area I want to tone up?

BAFTA bum

If you want to get the kind of toned, shapely bum which A-listers boast, the best exercises to do are squats and lunges, mixed with some running and skipping. At home, you can do step on your stairs – just take two steps at a time and squeeze your bum while you're doing it.

Bums have made people famous, and they can be every bit as important as having a beautiful face. Just think of J-Lo and Beyoncé. A backside can literally define someone, and celebs can build a career on a good bottom.

A-list arms

Arms are one of the most important parts of the body when it comes to looking toned. Boxing and light weight training are great if you want to achieve lean arms. Bigger weights will just bulk arms up. Dips are also good for toning the backs of your arms, which are the bane of so many women's lives. Arms are one of the things most susceptible to 'skinny fat'. They may be slender, but no celebrity wants their arms to start vibrating when they shake someone's hand on the red carpet.

Oscar abs

Everyone always assumes that sit-ups are the best exercise to do if you want to get a tight tummy. Not so. When you do sit-ups, you only really use two of the muscles in your stomach, and you're effectively ignoring all the muscles around them. While sit-ups are in no way bad, you need to work all the muscles in your stomach to get definition. Anything that makes you rotate your body is great, because it tones the muscles on the side of your stomach and helps to create that hourglass figure that we all love. If you look at pictures of old Roman soldiers, they always had amazing definition on their obliques – on the side of their stomachs – because they carried heavy swords and swung them around. That twisting movement creates definition.

Curls – which are also often called crunches – are also brilliant for stomach toning, as are reverse curls, where you lie on your back with your legs in the air and push your legs towards the ceiling as if you're kicking someone off you. They work your lower abs really well. If you want to mix it up, you can use a Swiss ball and do your exercises while you're watching TV.

A toned tummy not only looks good in a dress, but it makes you stand up straighter, giving the illusion of a slimmer frame.

BRITs back

Although it's not always practical and easy, kayaking and canoeing are excellent for toning up the stomach, and also the bits on your back which tend to sag. A sagging back is every celeb's worst nightmare, and it often gives away people's age, no matter how much facial surgery or Botox they've invested in.

If it's not practical for you to go canoeing (or you just don't fancy getting cold and wet – and who could blame you), there are also exercises you can do at home.

Anything that creates a pulling motion will help your back. Fill up a handbag with some heavy cans of food. Then whilst standing lean over so that your back is straight. Keep your back at a right angle and then pull your bag up and down so that your arms and upper back are doing most of the work. Next bend forward over the arm of the sofa so your head is facing the floor and, again, raise and lower a bag using one arm at a time. Do fifty raises on each side. Finally, you can lie on your front and pull up your head and arms – keeping your arms straight – as though you're flying. Then raise and lower your arms as many times as you can manage.

If you've got a kids' playground near you, the best things you can use are the monkey bars. You may have to build your strength up slowly in order to use them, but they will really benefit you.

Cannes Cans

There's nothing more annoying than spotting a gorgeous strapless dress only to try it on and watch in horror as your armpit flab – or 'chicken fillets', as they're often called – start creeping over the top of it. The best way to get rid of these is by doing press-ups, boxing and anything else that makes you do a pushing action. You can also try lying on the floor holding something heavy in each hand then pull your hands together and push them apart.

All of these exercises will strengthen the chest area and the muscles around your boobs, giving the illusion of a mini-uplift.

Get yourself some cheap tools

If you want to work out at home, there are some great, cheap pieces of equipment you can buy for £10 to £15:

- Skipping rope: this gives you a great cardio workout and helps to tone your bum.

- Trampet: this is a smaller version of a trampoline that you can use at home – you don't need lessons for this since you won't bounce much higher than half a foot!

- Dumb bells: fabulous for abs and arms.

- Swiss balls: can be used to tone most parts of your body.

- Abs and back exerciser: I think you can work this one out!

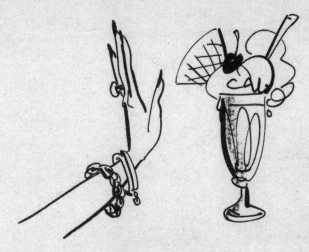

Chapter 8

What on earth does that mean? Why does that happen? And is that *really* true?

Why did I feel sick while I was exercising? (Warning: geeky science stuff)

Feeling sick when you are exercising is due to a build-up of lactic acid, which is a toxin in your blood. The by-product of this build-up of lactic acid is that you start to feel sick. And, if you pushed yourself that bit further, you may actually have vomited.

You need to know your limits – push yourself but not so hard that you feel ill. As you train, your threshold increases, so you can push yourself harder, as time goes on. It's all about building it up. Think of your threshold in terms of someone who has never drunk alcohol. If they go out and drink seven pints, the chances are they'll be very sick, because they have no tolerance for alcohol, and they won't be used to the toxins. But, if they carry on drinking over a few months, their threshold will become higher and, correspondingly, they'll be less likely to be sick. (Please note that we are in no way encouraging you to go out and train yourself to drink vast amounts of alcohol here – quite the opposite!)

So, basically, the fitter you are, and the more training you've done, the more tolerant you are of lactic acid. Rowers probably have one of the highest lactic-acid thresholds, because they have to work through it when they start to feel sick. They can't just stop in the middle of the water, so they have to learn to handle it and up their fitness levels to deal with it.

Luckily, the chances of you actually making yourself sick while you're training are incredibly low, unless you're ridiculously motivated and do not allow yourself to stop. If you do start to feel sick, take a break for a few minutes. The reason the lactic acid builds up is because the muscles are being used really fast but there isn't enough oxygen coming in. So, when you do get a chance to take in oxygen without using it all on exercise, that helps the blood flow through the muscles and disperses the lactic acid. That's why you warm down at the end of a training session – to get the oxygenated blood to your muscles in order to get rid of the lactic acid.

The worst thing you can do when you take a break is to bend over, which is what most people immediately do, because you're squashing your lungs and the oxygen won't be able to move round your body quickly enough. The best thing to do is to stand up straight, put your hands behind your head and take some deep breaths – just like runners do in the Olympics. And, if you can, carry on walking, even if it's slowly.

Your body needs time to cool down. It's far better to run and then walk (my clients always like the walking bit!), then run some more and walk some more, than run and stop dead. That way you'll reduce your heart rate to a comfortable level, and then, when you're ready, you can start running again.

My muscles ache – should I still exercise?

Yes, but make sure you use different parts of your body. If your arms are aching, work out using your legs. Nothing you do on this programme should make you ache so badly that you have to stop exercising for any length of time. Just vary it as much as possible.

Can I exercise with a hangover?

Definitely, it's the best thing you can possibly do. That's my cheat for beating a night out on the booze. If you exercise first thing, and drink plenty of water, it will stop you craving yellow foods such as bread and pastries – which is what most people tend to eat on a hangover, because they're stodgy and sweet – and it will help you get over your hangover far more quickly.

Obviously, in an ideal world, we'd all drink loads of water and eat two bananas before we go to bed to help flush the alcohol out and replace the vitamins we've lost to alcohol – but how often do we remember? A run is the next best thing. It will help you sweat out the toxins and clear your head.

Remember: it's not just the calories in the alcohol itself that makes you put on weight, it's the fact that you crave unhealthy foods the day after. A fry-up is traditionally seen as a hangover cure and, if you have one of those a couple of times a week, and a pizza or a kebab after a heavy night out, before you know it, you've put on weight.

A run will set you back on the straight and narrow and stop you wanting to eat fatty meals. Have a bowl of muesli, which is full of nutrients and will help your body to feel more balanced, and you'll soon be feeling fine again.

We all hear fitness terms bandied about, but what do they mean?

The thought of starting to exercise can be pretty intimidating in itself, without suddenly being confronted with all kinds of terms that completely go over your head. It's the feeling that fitness and training is almost another world that puts lots of people off. When it's been demystified, it suddenly seems a lot less scary. Our guide will help you get to grips with all that exercise terminology.

Aerobic exercise

Aerobic exercise is exercise that involves oxygen: for example, a low-intensity exercise that you do for a long time, such as a step class.

Cardiovascular exercise

This is very similar to aerobic training. Running, cycling and swimming are all cardiovascular.

Anaerobic exercise

These are exercises you do without the intake of oxygen. Sprinting is anaerobic. When you sprint a hundred metres, you don't actually need to breathe. For athletes, breathing is a waste of energy. It could make the difference between them winning a gold medal or not.

Dumb bell
This is a bar with weights on either side which you lift to help you tone up.

Circuit weight training
This is a series of linked exercises, generally working different muscles. The series can consist of anything from three to twenty exercises linked together.

Contraction
This is when the muscle contracts, or tenses.

Reps
This is the number of times you repeat each exercise in a session.

Resistance
This refers to the amount of weight that you're working against. For instance, if you're doing a push-up, your body is the weight of the resistance but, if you were weight lifting, the weight would be the resistance. So, if a dumb bell is 5kg, you're working with a 5kg resistance.

Target heart rate
This is the heart rate at which the fitness industry recommends you should be training. If you're trying to lose weight, it's recommended that you train at a certain

heart rate. If you're training to increase fitness, you train at a different heart rate.

Personally, I don't follow those rules. If you go on a cross trainer in a gym, you can fill in your age, weight, etc, and it gives a target heart rate. I think that, when people follow this to the letter, they start to develop pre-conceptions as to how hard they're going to be working before they've even got started. I've always found that I work harder when I don't use a target heart rate.

Maximum heart rate

This is the maximum rate your heart can function at, which is 220 minus your age.

Body-fat percentage

This refers to the percentage of your body that is made up of fat. People think that you can turn fat into muscle, but it's impossible to do that, because they're completely different substances. It would be like trying to turn a rusty old bike into a Ferrari. To lower body-fat percentage, you have to decrease fat as you increase muscle.

Endurance

This is the amount of time you can keep going – whether you're running, canoeing or lifting weights – before you get tired.

Fitness fact and fiction

- Calories are the main thing you need to worry about if you're trying to lose body fat.

False

Calories are basically a way of measuring how much energy you take in. If you take in a lot but burn more by doing training, the number of calories is irrelevant. It's your fat intake that you should be thinking about.

- Lifting lighter weights will make your muscles more defined and toned.

False

If you lift a light weight over and over again, it won't make your muscles grow bigger, and therefore lean and toned. In fact, it will take you forever to build any muscle at all.

You need to increase the size of the muscle to make it look good, and this just won't happen unless you use heavier weights. You won't end up with big, muscly, manly arms, (see above) but you do need to build up muscle to get rid of the fat on your arms.

- A woman will get huge arms if she lifts big weights.

False

Women have a third the amount of testosterone as men so, unless you're taking male hormones and steroids, it's going to take a woman a long, long time to build up big muscles.

- As you get older, you gain more fat and lose muscle – it's a fact of life.

False

Obviously, your metabolism slows down a bit but, as long as you stay in shape, you'll be fine. You can't use the excuse that it's your metabolism that's making you put on weight, because you can always do things to counteract it. This is where the maintenance part of the programme is worth its weight in gold since if you follow it you'll be able to keep your body in good working order and be in a much better position to avoid putting on weight.

- No pain, no gain

False

If I poked you in the arm with a spear, would you lose weight? No. Pain is just a by-product of working hard. Sometimes, you need to work hard, but you shouldn't put yourself through hell. If doing a workout were as easy and enjoyable as having a glass of wine, you'd never stop doing it. Unfortunately, that's not the case, but neither does exercise have to make you feel as if you have just been tortured for it to be doing you good. You need to find that all-important happy balance.

• Doing loads of cardio is the best way to lose body fat.

False

The best way to lose fat is to increase your muscle mass. That's why body-builders have the lowest body fat of any athletes.

• Muscles weigh more than fat.

True

Yes, they do. Obviously, if you compare a pound of fat and a pound of muscle, they're both going to weigh the same. But, volume to volume, muscle weighs three times more. This is something that's really good to remember for those times when your weight isn't dropping as quickly as you think it should be. Just because the scales aren't showing too much change, it doesn't mean that your body isn't getting into better shape.

- The best way to make a certain area look better is to concentrate on working on just that one particular part of your body.

False

You'll get much better results if you also tone up all the areas around it. For instance, if you wanted to get good abs, you could try sword fighting or canoeing, and you'll get much better results doing so, because you'll have worked other muscles that link in.

- You should never drink water while exercising.

False

You should *always* drink water. On a day when you're exercising, you should drink two more litres than normal, to rehydrate yourself and help eliminate toxins. It also helps to quicken your metabolism.

- If you're just doing fast walking, you don't have to worry about warming up or down.

False

You should always do some kind of warming up and down because whenever you're exerting your muscles there's a chance of injury.

- After a while your fitness levels and weight will plateau.

True

Yes, they will, but it's only temporary. If you keep training and following the diet, and changing your exercise routine, you will continue to improve.

- Vegetarians won't build muscles as well as people who eat meat.

False

Just because you're a vegetarian that doesn't hinder your ability to build muscle. Vegetarians can gain just as much protein from things such as cottage cheese, pulses, tofu and, if they eat it, fish, as they could from meat.

- The best time of the day to work out is in the morning.

False

There isn't a best time to work out – it's whatever is best for you. You just have to decide what will fit in with your lifestyle, so that you're less tempted to make excuses about not being able to do it and give up.

- As long as you're not planning to overdo it, you don't need to see your doctor before starting an exercise programme.

False

I would always recommend you see a doctor before you start any exercise programme. It will only take around twenty minutes.

- The more you exercise, the more protein you need to take in to maintain your energy levels.

False

Of the three types of nutrients – protein, fat and carbohydrates – protein actually provides the least energy, though it is very good for replenishing the muscles.

Diet facts and fiction

- Fad diets work.

False

No, no, no. You'll only end up putting on more weight afterwards, because you won't have lost weight sensibly. You'll still have a lot of fat in your body, so more fat will pile back on.

- Low-fat and non-fat foods don't have many calories.

False

Absolutely false. Calories and fat are two totally different things. Calories are the energy that you gain from eating the food, and fat is the actual fat that is in food. For instance, there's no fat in rice, but there are loads of calories, because it's a starchy carb and therefore pure energy. It's the same with pasta. At the same time, there's a certain amount of fat in salmon and meat, but not many calories. Another thing you have to watch out for with a lot of so-called 'diet foods' is that a lot of sugar and salt is added to make them taste nicer since, often, when the fat is stripped away, so is the flavour.

• Where you come from often has something to do with why you put on weight.

True

I believe that you may put weight on in different areas depending on which country you're from. Different nationalities do seem predisposed to particular types of weight gain. For instance, Italians always put on weight around their bellies.

I think that a lot of this is to do with the culture and history of each region or country. If you look back at British history, people who lived during famines ate lots of honey and fat, because they needed to take in the energy to work, and not a lot else was on offer. The rich people would eat lots of meat but, further down the social scale, the choice was far more limited. People couldn't afford to be picky eaters: if you didn't like the food on offer, you died. I think that maybe that's why we love fat and sugar so much.

The Japanese love their steamed rice and their fresh fish because that's all that was available during a famine. And the Greeks love olive oil, because it's remained a staple food when there wasn't a lot else around to eat. They still eat it a lot now, which is why a lot of Greeks put on weight – olive oil is very fattening. Obviously you shouldn't use this as an excuse for putting on weight, but it is worth bearing in mind.

• Eating late at night makes you put on weight.

True

Obviously, the earlier you eat, the more chance you have to burn the food off, especially carbs. This is why you should always weight your meals so that your most substantial food intake is breakfast, followed by a smaller portion at lunch, and less still at dinner. But, if you're eating something such as tomato soup or chicken, it doesn't make so much of a difference, because it's just protein which you can digest far more quickly than carboydrates.

• I can lose weight while eating whatever I want.

False

You can lose weight by eating cleverly, but no one in the world can eat three pizzas, four Thai takeaways and seven burgers in a week and still lose weight, even if they are exercising. The day someone does that, I will quit as a personal trainer. It's all about *what* you eat. Aside from this, if you're eating healthy food rather than something you've just called up from a fast-food restaurant, it's going to have a whole range of health benefits, on top of just losing weight.

- Fast foods are unhealthy and should be totally avoided when you're dieting.

False

Some fast foods can be healthy; it's a mistake to think that fast food is only about pizza and burgers. A chicken shish kebab with salad and no mayo is great – it's basically just a chicken salad. See the eating-out guide for more info.

- Dairy products are fattening and bad for you.

False

Some are. For instance, cheese and cream might be high in protein, but they're also very high in fat. However cottage cheese has no fat and is very good for you, and semi-skimmed milk is a great source of low-fat protein. Other good sources of protein where you don't need to take on fat at the same time are fish, lean meat and pulses such as chickpeas and lentils.

- Having a slow metabolism prevents weight loss.

False

So many people use this as an excuse for putting on weight, as if their metabolism was always at a fixed level. Yes, some people have a higher metabolic rate than others, but that doesn't mean you can't make your metabolism work for you. Exercise, eating regular meals and not overeating will all help keep your metabolism ticking over. Things such as green tea, water and grapefruit are also great for your metabolism.

- Eating red meat makes it harder to lose weight.

False

Red meat is fine as long as you're not eating it at every meal. Too much of anything is bad for you, but humans can digest fat and protein far more quickly than they can digest carbs. Red meat is also a great source of iron (which is the most common nutritional deficiency in the UK – especially for women), zinc and vitamin B.

- Vegetarians are healthier and lose weight much more easily.

False

Just because you stop eating meat, that doesn't make you any healthier. A lot of vegetarians eat lots of cheese and other high-fat foods instead. India has the largest vegetarian community in the world, but it also has the highest rate of heart disease on the planet. I was shocked when I found this out. That said, you should make a real effort to include as many vegetables as possible in your diet.

- No-fat diets are good for you

False

This opinion would be true if it was just referring to the kind of pre-packed low-fat foods available in the diet sections of the shops. They may well have a low fat content, but like all processed foods they tend to be packed with a whole list of other ingredients and preservatives which won't do your body any good at all. As with so much else of the programme, eating a low-fat diet is about common sense. If you fry all your food, or use lots of butter when cooking, then obviously your meals will not be as healthy. All nutritionists will tell you that you need to have a small amount of fat to maintain a balanced diet. However, if you want to become lean, then the less fat you take in, the easier this will be to achieve.

• If you give up smoking, you'll put on weight.

False

If you manage your metabolism and eat healthily, giving up smoking doesn't mean you have to put on weight. People do tend to snack more when they give up smoking (and this is more from force of habit than anything else), but they'll only put weight on if they always reach for a packet of crisps rather than snacking healthily. You need to remember that snacking isn't necessarily bad, it only becomes unhealthy if you eat the wrong things! Anyway, it's certainly not smoking itself that makes you slim – there are plenty of overweight people who smoke.

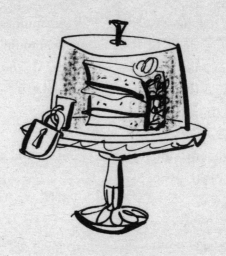

Chapter 9

And when you've finished . . . The essential maintenance bit

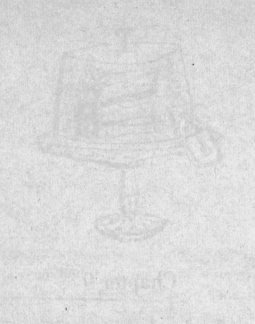

Because this diet isn't extreme, it is easy for you to carry on with it and integrate it into your everyday life. I could have made it much more extreme, but I know that, if I were to do that, the weight you have lost would go back on quickly, like it does with fad diets.

By the time you've finished the plan, you will have re-educated yourself about food, and you'll know what will and what won't put weight on. It's about achieving that all-important balance.

If you want to carry on losing weight, continue with the plan as you have been. If you just want to maintain your weight, you can reintroduce some carbs into your everyday diet – but don't go from nothing to everything. If you're going to eat carbs, have them for breakfast or lunch, so that you give your body the chance to burn them off during the day. For instance, don't snack on a huge sandwich before you go to bed, because your body won't have any time to use up the energy it provides.

By the end of the six weeks, you will have learned how many alternatives there are to carbs when it comes to breakfast, lunch and dinner, so there won't be any need for you to have toast for breakfast, sandwiches for lunch and pasta for dinner. Be sensible about it: there's no need to give up on everything you've learned once you've finished the plan and immediately revert to bad habits.

It stands to reason that, if you start eating fatty food again every day, you will start putting some of the weight you've lost back on – albeit more slowly than you would have done in the past, now that your body is leaner, more muscular and, crucially, more efficient – so make sensible choices and remember how good you're feeling about yourself right now.

A great way to maintain your new, lower weight is to plan way ahead. You can literally take the next year into account, earmarking any big events you've got coming up, and set yourself targets.

If Easter is rolling around, and you know you're going to be tempted to eat loads of chocolate, cut down on sugary or fattening foods and up your exercise in the run-up to it so you can enjoy an egg and a hot cross bun knowing that you've factored it in.

If you've got a wedding to go to, it's going to be

practically impossible to sit there with everyone else and not eat what they're eating, so plan to go for a run or do some other exercise the following day to counteract any unhealthy foods you eat.

Manage your year, as opposed to doing it week by week. If you know you've got a holiday planned, make time to do more exercise and cut down on carbs for a couple of months beforehand. That way, you can lose a few pounds, and you'll be able to enjoy food and drink while you're away, without panicking about putting on weight.

By setting yourself goals, you always have something to aim towards, and you know when you can take things easier, and when you need to be stricter with yourself. Dip in and out and work the plan around your job, going out and your holidays.

The trick is to give yourself a buffer zone. If you're usually around ten stone, but you feel your best at nine and a half stone, give yourself a zone of between nine and a half and ten and a half stone, and make sure you always stay within that. It's absolutely not about yo-yo dieting; it's simply about working harder when you want to look leaner.

Obviously, once you've finished the six weeks, it is totally up to you as to how closely you decide to follow the plan from then on. But, if you want some basic rules to follow long term, here they are:

- Keep cheese and cream to a minimum. It's no secret that they're packed with fat.

- Sugar is the biggest evil. Sugar doesn't give you anything good. It gives you a big high, but it also gives you a big low. It makes things taste good, but you get addicted to it. It's like a bad boyfriend – it will never make you happy.

- Avoid sweeteners. Sweeteners are the same as sugar, but what is in them is even worse for you. If you're going to eat sugar or take sweeteners, believe it or not, I would rather you ate sugar. The by-products contained in sweeteners are the same as those used to preserve organs in museums. Do you really want that floating around your body?

- Stay away from diet products. These contain so many additives, and they're so processed, that they're hard for your body to break down. Often, they also contain loads of sweeteners (see above). It's a million times better for you to prepare your own foods. It may take a bit longer, but the health benefits are ten times better. Generally, healthy people cook for themselves. And cooking is fun.

- Avoid carbs in the evening. If you eat a load of carbs in the evening and then go to sleep, you don't work them off with exercise, so those fats will stick to your belly. If you eat and then go for a run before you turn in, then fine but, unsurprisingly, very few people want to do that . . .

- Only drink alcohol twice a week. I know I talk about alcohol a lot, but it's one of the easiest ways to put and keep weight on, especially because you always want to eat unhealthy foods that night and the next day. Apart from being fun, alcohol has no positive benefits, and it's too easy to get into a pattern of sitting down to enjoy a glass of wine each night. Those calories build up quickly, and can be the difference between your skinny jeans fitting and not fitting. People think because it's not food you won't put on weight. Sadly, they're wrong.

- Train twice a week. Come on, it's not hard.

- Stop eating when you're full. Even if you're eating healthy foods, be aware of how you're feeling and, once you start to feel full, stop. Years of dieting often leave people veering between not eating much and then clearing everything on their plate, just because they can. It actually takes twenty minutes for your brain to register that your stomach is full, so eat slowly and enjoy your food; don't stuff it down. You'll only end up feeling uncomfortable and giving yourself a hard time about it. There's nothing to prevent you eating more later, so stop if you think you're getting full and, if you're still hungry in half an hour, eat again.

- Don't skip meals. You may be lowering your calorie intake, but you're also slowing down your metabolism, because you're not keeping it burning correctly. So your metabolism will lower and burn fat at a slower rate, and then, when you eat a lot of food, it's trying to go from zero to a hundred miles an hour, and that will never work.

- Treat yourself. If you totally deny yourself things, you could end up going the other way and eating loads of rubbish. If you want something, have it. Just don't have loads of it, and don't have it every day. If you want a few nuts or some chocolate, have them. Just don't have a bag of nuts, and then a huge bar of chocolate, and then some cake. When things are a treat and not an everyday occurrence, you appreciate them so much more.

Have you ever gone on holiday and, on the first day, you've gone for it and drunk absolutely loads?

Then, by the fourth day, you don't know how you'll ever drink again, because you've overdone it and taken away all the enjoyment? It's the same with treats. If you have them all the time, you take away the true enjoyment of them. By having them less often, you'll appreciate them so much more. If you had a friend, or a boyfriend, you saw every second of every day, you'd probably get bored with them and be desperate for a break. But if you didn't see them that often, you'd probably really look forward to seeing them and cherish the time you spent with them.

It's the same with anything. When I was a kid, I loved basketball, and I used to play every day for hours, any chance I got. Then, when I was sixteen, I turned professional, and someone started paying me for it and telling me when I had to do it. A couple of years in, it stopped being fun. But, now, I miss it, because no one is trying to force me to do it.

Food is no different. If you overload yourself with certain foods, it takes away the excitement and the fun of them, and eating them becomes more of a habit rather than being something you really appreciate.

Follow these rules, and you'll keep your weight off, and will probably even lose some more. Don't view it as a diet, though; view it as a healthy lifestyle. It takes the pressure off, and makes you feel as if you're being good to yourself and looking after your body, rather than depriving yourself. You deserve to look and feel good, and this will help you do that – in the long term. The recipes at the end of the book are here to help you maintain your healthy lifestyle (and keep your great new body) whilst still allowing you to enjoy eating as much you did before starting the plan.

This is a lifestyle plan, and these things will eventually just become a part of your everyday life, like brushing your teeth. If you didn't brush your teeth, they would rot, and you'd have bad breath. Just as you have to treat your teeth right, so you have to do the same with your body. If you don't eat healthily and exercise, you're going to be unfit and put on weight.

Wake up in the morning and go for a quick jog. On Monday night, when you get home and you're craving a bottle of wine, stop yourself. But, the next night, go out with the girls and party if you want to. It's all about balance.

Here are some stories to keep you motivated:

Boot-camp beauty

One lady who came on my boot camp last year had been trying to lose weight for years. She was carrying a stubborn stone and a half, which wouldn't shift, no matter what she did.

She wanted to come on the boot camp to learn about nutrition and to find out which exercises worked for her, which is exactly what she did. She could easily have gone back, patted herself on the back for having worked so hard when she was at the camp and returned to her normal eating habits.

However, when she got back home, she discovered that she'd lost four pounds, and that was all the encouragement she needed to stick with what she'd learned. She continued the programme, ate sensibly and joined a gym, where she found she loved doing spinning classes.

I had an email from her six weeks later, in which she very proudly told me that she had lost another stone and was fitting back into jeans she hadn't been able to wear for fifteen years.

The plan totally changed her life, and she now maintains it by following the rules of eating good food, exercising two to three times a week and only drinking twice a week – which is pretty impressive, as she is the manageress of a bar.

She's managed to fit the plan into her life rather

than having to plan her life around it. It's second nature to her now and, if she does have a big night out, she doesn't give herself a hard time, she just works a bit harder in the gym next time around.

She admits that she has the odd week when it's really difficult to stick to the rules because of work commitments or holidays or whatever, but she's learned that it doesn't mean she needs to give up everything altogether and ruin all the hard work she's put in to get to her goal weight.

As she said, 'I worked so hard to lose that weight, so why would I allow it to go back on in a matter of weeks? It doesn't make sense. For me, it's all about getting the balance right, and if I'm not great for a week, I'm a lot better the next week. I've got a life, the same as everyone else, but I also know that I never want to be unhappy with how I look again.'

Revenge is sweet

A girl in her thirties came to me a few years ago, because she'd been dumped by her boyfriend in quite a horrible way two months earlier. Because she was miserable, all she'd done was eat, and she'd gone from a size 10 to a size 16. She was still a very pretty girl, but she just didn't feel good about herself.

A few sessions in, she started to look much healthier and happier, and she could feel things changing. After a couple of months or so, she was down to a size 12, her self-esteem had improved and she was starting to date again.

She met one guy, and was starting to fall for him when, all of a sudden, her ex-boyfriend got wind of the fact she was seeing someone and got back in touch, saying he wanted to see her. She put off meeting up with him, but a month and a half later, he was still hassling her, so she decided she had to see him. When she turned up, she was looking incredible, and he immediately asked her to go out with him again, but she turned him down.

She called me three months later to tell me that her ex-boyfriend wouldn't leave her alone and had even proposed, but she'd continued to turn him down, and she was marrying the other guy.

I went to their wedding a year ago, and she admitted to me that, if she hadn't started exercising, she would have carried on eating and eating, and would have ended up alone and very unhappy – and not because no one would have fancied her when she was at her bigger size, but because she wouldn't have had the self-confidence to go out and meet anyone. She's now quit her job, moved to New York and become a personal trainer, and she's never been happier.

Detox disaster

I had a client who went on a detox. She lost just under two stone in two weeks, because she was on a juice-only diet and didn't eat anything, let alone drink any alcohol. By the time she came to me six weeks later, she had put it all back on – and then some.

She had been trying to lose the weight again, but she'd barely been eating, so her metabolism had slowed right down. I increased the amount she was eating, packed her diet full of healthy foods and allowed her to drink twice a week, and she started training four times a week. Within three months, she lost two and a half stone and, this time, she's kept it off. She couldn't believe she could drink champagne and eat food and still lose weight. She still does now, and none of the weight has gone back on.

Bye-bye yo-yo

A girl in her twenties who was a size ten came to me. She didn't want to lose any more weight, but she wanted to tone up. She kept her figure by barely eating anything but, every now and again, she would fall off the wagon, eat badly and put on weight. Then she would simply diet back to a size 10 and start the process all over again.

During our sessions, I re-educated her about eating and exercise, and now she keeps her size-10 figure without having to diet. If she falls off the wagon every now and again – as we all do – she does some exercise, and then she feels good about herself. She no longer sees it as a grand failure, and doesn't panic that she's ruined all her good work. She's learned to strike that all-important balance.

As she says, 'It's amazing that my weight doesn't fluctuate any more. I know it sounds crazy, but it's given me a real sense of freedom. I have takeaways, I go out with my mates and I don't feel as if I need to worry. Exercise doesn't feel like a chore, because I know it's doing me good and, weirdly, I actually enjoy it now. My friends are convinced someone else has taken over my body, but they can see how happy I am.'

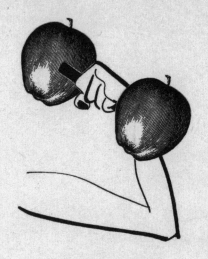

Chapter 10

Case study:
Sarah's been there and
done it – here's her story

Thirty-two-year-old Sarah from south-west London had tried every diet and exercise plan going when she came to see me for training. As soon as she heard about the Red Carpet Workout, she was desperate to try it, and she kindly agreed to keep a weekly diary charting her progress. Here's how she got on.

I must have tried every diet going over the past ten years or so, including drinking smoothies, or shakes, and only eating eggs for days on end (yes, really). I've also been through loads of phases with exercise, where I've gone to the gym continuously for weeks on end, and then not been again for two years. I think it's safe to say I'm an all-or-nothing girl.

I had always been fairly slim, until I went to university, but three years of cheap beer and takeaways took their toll, and I came home three stone heavier than I went, weighing in at twelve and a half stone. I soon set about trying to lose the weight, as I was planning to move to London and get a job, and I wanted to feel confident and happy with myself.

The first two stone came off pretty easily but, sadly, that last stone has stuck with me pretty much ever since. I've got down to my pre-uni weight of nine and a half stone several times, only to see my weight creep back up as soon as I quit whichever ridiculous diet I'm favouring at the time.

I now spend most of my time hovering between 10 stone 5lb and 10 stone 9lb, and I'm desperate to lose that excess stone and keep it off for good. I'm bored with waking up worrying about which of my clothes will still fit me, and then mulling over which of the fifteen or so diets I've done before I should try again.

As soon as I met Joe, he explained to me that, in order to lose the weight and keep it off permanently, I would need to combine healthy eating with exercise and lose the pounds slowly and sensibly (something which I have never managed before – I tend to panic and go for the quick-fix option). As soon as Joe told me about the premise of the Red Carpet Workout, it made perfect sense. As he said, there's no great mystery about losing weight, you just need to do it the right way.

I must admit, it's been a couple of years since I did

any exercise, so the thought of popping on my trainers and pounding the pavements is quite scary, but I used to get a real high from exercise, and Joe assures me that it won't take me too long to get back into it and build up my stamina. Hmmm, we'll see ...

As it's been a while since I exercised, I'm going to follow the Lazy Girl workout, and then upgrade later to the Savvy Girl workout if I make good progress!

Week 1

Monday

I did my first run today before work (I'm a marketing executive for a big American company and I have to be in at 8.30 every morning so, believe me, that was early) and, while I did have to do a lot of walking in between, I managed to go round the block three times without feeling as if I was going to collapse.

I'm going to take it slow and see everything I do as a small achievement rather than putting myself under huge pressure. I know what I'm like – if something is too hard, or I'm not enjoying it, I'll want to give up immediately.

I felt pretty good after my run and, when I got back home, I weighed myself and recorded my starting weight – 10 stone 6lb. If I can lose half a stone on the plan, I'll be happy.

I've already been shopping and bought in plenty of meat, salad and vegetables so, after a breakfast of muesli, I made myself a chicken and red pepper salad to take to work. I'm lucky, because there are fridges that I can store food in, which will make things much easier over the coming weeks.

Tuesday

I'm resisting the temptation to jump on the scales after just one day, even though I feel that, after my healthy eating yesterday, I must have lost some weight! I was feeling a bit groggy this morning, so I decided against a run, and I may try and go for one after work this evening, or see if one of my friends wants to come to the park with me. I do feel better exercising with a friend.

I'm having yoghurt for breakfast, and I've got some leftover turkey and vegetable curry that I made for dinner last night, so I'm going to take that to work for lunch. I've got quite a bad sugar craving, as I didn't touch a morsel yesterday, but I'm going to battle through it.

Wednesday

Okay, hands up: the run didn't happen last night. I was tired when I got in from work, so I had steak and vegetables and slobbed out in front of the TV. I am, however, playing netball tonight. My friend Lou has been hassling me for ages to join her team, and now I'm going to. I used to love it when I was younger so, hopefully, it will feel as if I'm exercising without actually exercising, if you see what I mean.

I'm still getting quite bad sugar cravings, and I'm missing my morning coffee and daytime tea, but I keep telling myself how good I'll feel once the cravings pass.

Breakfast today is two poached eggs, lunch is going to be chicken skewers (from the café over the road, as I don't have time to make them) and dinner will be whatever is in the fridge when I get back from netball.

I'm still managing to stop myself getting the scales out, on Joe's insistence, but I'm hopeful that I'll already have lost a couple of pounds. But maybe I'm just being a bit overly optimistic.

Thursday

It turns out that I'm still very good at netball. Who knew? Lou has asked me if I want to play every week, so I'm going to count that as one of my forms of exercise, which is allowed in the plan. So I only have one more exercise session to do this week, which is definitely doable.

Friday

I gave in yesterday and had some chocolate. I know it's a bit soon to be using my wild card, but someone brought jumbo-sized bars of Green & Blacks into the office, and it was too hard to resist, because my chocolate cravings were reaching fever pitch.

I only had a few squares, though, and then managed to stop myself going crazy, so I don't feel too bad. And I did get up and do my run today, which means that I now have my entire weekend free to chill out, albeit it without my usual takeaway and wine in front of the TV.

The food side of things is going well, though, and I made a huge tuna salad last night, so the rest is coming to work with me today for lunch.

Saturday

Oh dear. I popped out for one after-work drink last night and ended up having several. I stuck to champagne, as Joe instructed, but I didn't feel great when I woke up this morning, it has to be said. So I did something that I never in my life thought I would do – I went for a run. Joe had insisted that if anything will get rid of a hangover, it's a swift jog, but I honestly expected to give up after a couple of minutes and walk meekly back to my flat. But it actually works. I felt so much better when I got home and, after a hot shower,

I was able to go and meet my friends for lunch in a gastro pub in Greenwich.

I'm lucky that all my friends are being supportive, because it wouldn't have taken much encouragement for me to order the sticky toffee pudding and custard. Instead, I had a chicken breast marinated in chilli and ginger for my main, which was absolutely delicious.

Sunday

It's weigh-in day. I can't wait any longer. I was going to try and leave it until the middle of next week, but I'm glad I didn't, as I've lost three pounds in the first seven days, which has definitely given me the drive to carry on. I don't think I look much different when I stand in front of the mirror, but I definitely feel less bloated.

My sugar and caffeine cravings have all but gone, and I've definitely got a bit more energy too – although I'm not about to go out and start running marathons or anything just yet.

Weight loss in week 1: 3lb. Yay!

Week 2

Surprisingly, week 2 has been harder for me than week 1. Even though I was feeling really motivated by my weight loss, my friends and I all went for a curry on Tuesday night for a birthday celebration, and it was so hard not tucking into the naan breads and beer. But I did feel better for it the next day.

I went to netball again, and also went to the local gym a couple of times to use the free weights and have a run (it's been raining all week, so the thought of going round the block didn't really appeal), and now I'm not going out drinking as much as I was, it's a lot easier to fit everything in. I used to be a good four-nights-out-a-week kind of girl, but I've cut it down to two for the plan.

Foodwise, things have been pretty good. My cravings and headaches have disappeared, and I've been feeling so much better that I actually haven't wanted to touch sugar or caffeine at all.

I tried on a pair of my old jeans on Saturday, and they're definitely slightly looser, and my muffin top seems smaller. I'm also convinced that I can feel a muscle or two in my arms, but that may be just wishful thinking.

Weight loss in week 2: 1lb. A bit disappointing, but I can still see a slight difference in my body.

Week 3

I'm on a roll. I managed four lots of exercise this week – netball, a run, and I also went for two bike rides with my friend Clare. She's always told me how great cycling is, but I've never really been into the idea, but I found that it was good fun, even if I did have to be careful of dodgy London drivers. I also did some of the BAFTA Bum exercises in my living room, as I really want to tone up that area.

I've had three nights out this week, but I only drank on two of them, and then only a few vodkas each time. It's quite refreshing not waking up with hangovers all the time, and my head feels clearer than it has done in ages. I've also noticed that my eyes look shinier, and one of my workmates told me the other day that I was looking surprisingly healthy, which I guess means that I didn't look very healthy before starting the plan.

The weekend has been quite tough, as Saturday was a really miserable day and I was craving comfort food, but as soon as I had lunch (turkey breast with vegetables with a spicy tomato sauce), I stopped thinking about it.

Weight loss in week 3: 1lb. It's not loads, but
it means I've lost five pounds in all, which
Joe told me is a healthy and steady weight

loss. It also means I'm near my half-stone goal.

Week 4

I'm over halfway now, which feels amazing. Some parts of this week have been a bit tough, as I had a friend's wedding to go to and was dreading not being able to do my usual 'drinking all day' trick. But then, when I put my dress on and it was loose on me, I remembered why I was doing all this and I almost burst into tears.

It's the first time I've properly noticed how different my body looks. The last time I tried the dress on, it was very snug around my hips and bottom, but it now slips on no problem, and I got several compliments during the day. I also managed to have several glasses of champagne but not go too crazy (I felt very smug the next morning when all of my friends were feeling terrible), and I used my wild card to have some delicious chocolate wedding cake. I won't lie – it was amazing – but it didn't send me spiralling into a two-day chocolate binge or anything. I just saw it as a treat and got straight back on the plan on Sunday.

Exercise-wise I've been cycling, for a run and also played netball, so I did one session less than last week, but I still feel proud. I've been doing toning exercises at home in the evenings, and I can exercise for a lot longer without taking a break now. I can definitely see more definition in my arms and legs, which feels brilliant.

> Weight loss in week 4: 2lb. I've lost half a stone, and I can't believe I've reached my goal already. I feel amazing; not just in terms of weight loss, but energy-wise too. And only two more weeks to go. Sticky toffee pudding, here I come.

Week 5

Somehow, I ended up exercising five times this week, which is all a bit of a shock. I actually found myself wanting to go to the gym, and I also played netball and went for another bike ride with Clare. I think because there are only two weeks left, I feel as if I want to really go for it and make the most of it. I've also done the A-list Arms and BAFTA Bum exercises at home a few times, and my backside feels as if it's lifted a bit, which it certainly needed to.

This has been the easiest week so far. I don't know why, but I'm guessing I've just got into a bit of a routine. Foodwise, things have been great. I've very quickly learned that I don't have to live on lettuce leaves and, when a friend suggested dinner the other night, we went for sushi, and there was loads I could eat.

The plan isn't affecting my social life anywhere near as much as I thought it would, because I can still drink on it, and getting up and going for a run the next morning clears my head pretty swiftly, so it doesn't mean I'm glued to the sofa or falling asleep over my keyboard the following day.

I won't deny that there are some things I miss. The chocolate counter is always cruelly positioned exactly where you have to pay in shops, and it's an ongoing battle not to throw a bar or two into my basket. But then I realize that it would be pointless to cheat as – pardon the terrible cliché – I'm only going to be cheating myself. And the more people comment on how well I'm looking (read: there aren't chubby bits hanging over the top of my skirt any more), the more I feel motivated to carry on.

Weight loss in week 5: 2lb. Nine pounds in all. Wow.

Week 6

It's the last week. I'm so excited. I keep picturing all the foods I want to eat once it's all over. Needless to say, a big bar of chocolate is at the top of my list, as well as that much-talked-about sticky toffee pudding.

I've been to the gym four times, done the Oscar Abs, etc, exercises at home several times, and I've also been cycling. There was no netball this week, but I'm going to go back next week, even though I'll have finished the plan. I've started to love it, and I think I would really miss it if I stopped now.

The only problem was that, instead of playing netball, some of the team went out for drinks on Wednesday, and I was no exception. I managed to stick to vodka, soda water and fresh lime, but I wasn't quite as good when we all went for a Chinese afterwards. I felt very saintly ordering my stir-fried vegetables, but as soon as Lou offered me some of her special fried rice, I scooped some on to my plate. I hadn't used my wild card at all this week, so I decided that I would use it then. And I didn't fall off the wagon for the rest of the week, so it wasn't the end of the world.

I tried on the jeans I wore in week 2 again, and the waist is literally falling off me. They look so big now that I'm not even sure that I can wear them any more. I'm planning a shopping trip for some new ones next weekend. I must have saved a fortune on going out over the past six weeks, so I feel totally justified in splashing out on some new clothes to say a big well done to myself.

I honestly didn't think I'd make it through the whole six weeks, but I feel so proud of myself. I've lost count of the number of people who have told me that I look well and, when I bumped into an ex-boyfriend from a few years ago last week, he was extremely flirty with me. And while I'm not in the least bit interested, it was just the boost I needed, especially seeing as he was the one who dumped me!

Weight loss in week 6: 2lb. I've lost eleven pounds in total, and I feel better than I have in years. I won't deny that there were times when I wanted to fast track the weight loss and wished I could drop five pounds in a week, but I know that, this way, there's much less chance of it going straight back on again. It's all been so worth it, and much easier than I imagined it would be. Now, where's the nearest cake shop . . .

2 weeks later

Despite expecting myself to run out and throw down lashings of wine and fattening foods, in the week after I finished the plan, I found myself actually wanting to stick with it. I did falter here and there and, yes, I did have the sticky toffee pudding I promised myself, but I've kept up with the exercise and have kept carbs to a minimum, and I've now lost nearly a stone.

I'm definitely going to carry on following the maintenance part of the plan, as much for my energy levels and how good I feel as anything else. I love having more energy, and I'm certainly not willing to slip back into my old, bad habits.

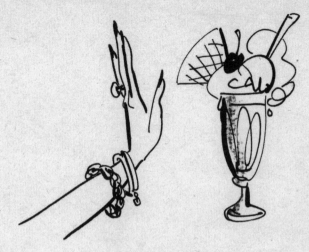

Chapter 11

For those of you who don't use your oven to store shoes ... here are some recipes

Now that you have achieved your goal and have a fabulous, healthy, new lifestyle, why not impress your friends by inviting them round for a delicious dinner? But, remember: although these recipes are devised to be low in fat, salt and calories and high in nutrients, they're intended to help keep your body in shape after you've finished the plan rather than help you lose weight during it.

Chicken, bacon and cheese kebabs

Serves 4

Preparation and cooking time: 20–25 minutes

4 skinless chicken breast fillets, about 175g (6oz) each
juice of 2 large lemons
salt and freshly ground black pepper
16 rashers lean bacon
115g (4oz) Gruyère cheese
24 cherry tomatoes
olive-oil spray
handful fresh herbs, such as flat-leaf parsley, coriander or basil, roughly chopped, to garnish

Preheat the grill to medium hot. Cut each chicken breast into eight bite-sized pieces and place in a bowl with the lemon juice. Season to taste with salt and pepper, toss to mix well and set to one side.

Remove all visible fat from the bacon and cut each rasher into two long strips. Cut the cheese into 32 even-sized chunks.

Place a chunk of cheese on top of each piece of chicken, then wrap together with a strip of bacon.

Take eight metal kebab skewers and alternately push four bacon-wrapped chicken-and-cheese pieces and three cherry tomatoes on to each skewer. Spray lightly with olive oil.

Place the skewers under the hot grill (or over the hot coals of a barbecue) for 8–10 minutes, turning once, or until the chicken is cooked through (any juices from the chicken should be clear, with no trace of blood).

Serve immediately, sprinkled with some of the roughly chopped fresh herbs, accompanied by a mixed-leaf salad.

Variations:
If you're not in the mood for chicken, try using chunks of fresh cod or another firm, white fish instead.

If you don't fancy tomatoes, strips of red, yellow or green pepper, onion wedges or chunks of courgette make delicious alternatives.

Add an Italian twist by using Parma ham rather than bacon.

Tuna ratatouille

Serves 4

Preparation and cooking time: 25–30 minutes

4 fresh tuna steaks, about 115g (4oz) each
salt and freshly ground black pepper
olive-oil spray
3 medium onions, finely chopped
4 cloves garlic, finely chopped
2 red peppers, deseeded and thickly sliced
4 medium courgettes, roughly chopped
2 medium aubergines, roughly chopped
2 x 400g (14oz) tins chopped tomatoes
1 tsp sugar
1 tbsp dried mixed herbs
large handful fresh, flat-leaf parsley, roughly chopped

Season the tuna steaks lightly with salt and pepper and set to one side.

Heat a large pan or wok over a medium heat and spray lightly with olive oil. Add the onion and garlic, and cook for 2–3 minutes. Toss in the peppers, courgettes and aubergines, stir and cook for a further 3–4 minutes. Stir in the chopped tomatoes, sugar and mixed herbs, and season to taste with salt and pepper. Lower the heat and leave to bubble gently for 6–8 minutes, or until the vegetables are just tender.

Meanwhile, spray the tuna steaks lightly with olive oil. Heat a ridged griddle pan (or frying pan) until very hot. Add the tuna to the pan and cook for 2–3 minutes on each side, until just cooked through (it should still be slightly pink in the middle).

Divide the cooked vegetables between four warm serving plates. Top each plate with a freshly cooked tuna steak and serve immediately, sprinkled with a garnish of freshly chopped parsley.

Rosemary and garlic lamb with spring onion mash

Serves 4

Preparation and cooking time: 35–40 minutes

4 x 250–300g (9–10½oz) racks of lamb (ask your butcher to trim off most of the fat, or buy ready-trimmed from a supermarket)
olive-oil spray
5 large cloves garlic
10–12 large sprigs fresh rosemary, finely chopped

salt and freshly ground black pepper
900g (2lb) butternut squash
bunch of spring onions, finely chopped
6–8 tbsp very low-fat fromage frais

Preheat the oven to 190ºC (375ºF, Gas 5). Place the racks of lamb on a baking tray, rib side up. Using a small, sharp knife, make slashes all over the meat and spray lightly with olive oil.

Peel the garlic and, using a pestle and mortar, crush to a paste. Mix in the chopped rosemary and then spread the mixture evenly over the meat. Season well with salt and pepper and bake in the hot oven for 25–30 minutes, or until cooked to your liking.

While the meat is cooking, peel and dice the butternut squash and cook in a pan of boiling, lightly salted water for 15 minutes, or until tender. Drain and mash until smooth. Stir in the spring onions and fromage frais, and season to taste with salt and pepper. If necessary, re-heat the mash and serve with the freshly cooked lamb, accompanied by steamed greens or a leafy salad.

Seafood stir-fry with vegetable tagliatelle

Serves 4

Preparation and cooking time: 20–25 minutes

2 medium carrots, peeled
2 medium courgettes, trimmed
olive-oil spray
1 medium onion, sliced
2 cloves garlic, finely chopped
2½cm (1in) piece fresh ginger, peeled and finely chopped
1 red pepper, deseeded and thinly sliced
1 yellow pepper, deseeded and thinly sliced
800g (1lb 12oz) mixed seafood
handful each fresh mint and coriander, roughly chopped
salt and freshly ground black pepper

Using a vegetable peeler or mandolin, cut the carrots and courgettes into long, thin strands to resemble tagliatelle pasta. Plunge into a pan of boiling water for 1–2 minutes, drain, set to one side and keep warm.

Heat a wok or large frying pan over a high heat. Spray lightly with olive oil, add the onion and stir-fry for

3–4 minutes, or until soft. Toss in the garlic and ginger and stir-fry for a further 30 seconds, then add the sliced peppers and seafood. Continue to stir-fry the mixture for 3–4 minutes, until the peppers have softened and the seafood has warmed through. Remove from the heat, stir in the chopped mint and coriander and season to taste with salt and pepper.

Divide the vegetable tagliatelle between four warmed serving bowls, top with the stir-fry seafood and vegetable mixture and serve immediately.

Warm lentil salad with poached eggs and crispy bacon

Serves 4

Preparation and cooking time: 40–45 minutes

325g (11½oz) Puy lentils (Puy lentils have a delicious nutty taste and remain firm after cooking, but any type of lentil can be used)
olive-oil spray
1 medium red onion, roughly chopped
2 medium carrots, diced
2 celery stalks, diced
350g (12oz) cherry tomatoes

large handful flat-leaf parsley, roughly chopped
5 tbsp fat-free vinaigrette
salt and freshly ground black pepper
4 eggs
350g (12oz) lean bacon rashers
1–2 tbsp quark

Place the lentils in a large saucepan. Add enough cold water to cover, bring to the boil, reduce the heat and cook gently for 25–30 minutes, or until the lentils are just tender. Drain, set to one side and keep warm.

Heat a wok or large frying pan until hot. Spray lightly with olive oil, add the onion and stir-fry for 3–4 minutes, or until soft. Add the carrots, celery and tomatoes and stir-fry for a further 3–4 minutes, or until the vegetables are just tender and the mixture is warmed through. Add the lentils to the vegetables and stir to mix well. Remove from the heat and stir in the freshly chopped parsley and vinaigrette. Season to taste with salt and pepper, set to one side and keep warm.

Poach the eggs in gently simmering water until just cooked, and grill the bacon until crispy, and then dice. Divide the lentil salad between four warm serving bowls, top each bowl with a poached egg, scatter over the bacon and, finally, dot each serving with a teaspoon or two of quark. Serve immediately.

Baked salmon with spinach and broccoli

Serves 4

Preparation and cooking time: 40 minutes

4 x 175g (6oz) salmon fillets
2 tbsp olive oil
1 tbsp lemon juice
¼ tsp salt
¼ tsp black pepper
1 tbsp ground flaxseed
1 clove garlic, finely chopped
olive-oil spray
450g (1lb) fresh spinach
250g (9oz) broccoli

Preheat the oven to 230°C (450°F, Gas 8). Place the salmon fillets in a large dish. Mix the olive oil, lemon juice, salt, pepper, flaxseed and garlic together well in a small bowl and pour over the fish to coat it. Cover and leave in the fridge for at least 30 minutes.

Line a baking sheet with foil and spray lightly with olive oil. Remove the fish from the marinade and place it skin side down on the oiled foil on the baking sheet. Pour over any marinade remaining in the dish and bake in the hot oven for 9–12 minutes.

While the fish is cooking, lightly steam the spinach and broccoli until just tender. To serve, divide the vegetables between four warm serving plates. Top with a piece of cooked salmon and serve immediately.

Chicken chow mein

Serves 4

Preparation and cooking time: 40–45 minutes

1 tbsp sunflower oil
225g (8oz) skinless chicken breast fillets
175g (6oz) medium egg noodles – dry weight
1 medium onion, thinly sliced
2½cm (1in) piece fresh ginger, peeled and thinly sliced
2 cloves garlic, thinly sliced
175g (6oz) fresh beansprouts
175g (6oz) mangetout, trimmed
1 tsp five-spice powder
2 tbsp dark soy sauce

Preheat the oven to 190°C (375°F, Gas 5).

Put a piece of foil (approximately 30 x 40cm/12 x 16in) on to a baking sheet and brush with a little (approximately 1 teaspoon) of the oil.

Place the chicken breasts side by side in the middle of the foil and sprinkle over about two tablespoons of water. Close the foil around the chicken to make a loose, but tightly closed, parcel. Bake in the hot oven for 30–35 minutes, until the chicken is cooked through (any juices from the meat should run clear, with no sign of blood). Remove the chicken from the oven; allow it to cool slightly, shred and set to one side.

Cook the noodles in a large pan of boiling, salted water, according to the instructions on the packet.

While the noodles are cooking, heat a wok or large frying pan over a high heat, add the remaining oil, then add the onion and ginger and stir-fry for 2–3 minutes, or until the onion softens. Add the garlic, beansprouts, mangetout and five-spice powder and continue stir-frying for another minute.

Drain the cooked noodles well and add to the wok or frying pan. Toss in the shredded chicken and soy sauce.

Stir-fry for a further 2 minutes until piping hot. Serve immediately.

Hot Thai beef salad

Serves 4

Preparation and cooking time: 1 hour 15 minutes

450g (1lb) sirloin steak, cut into thin strips,
approximately 7½cm (3in) long and ½cm (¼in) wide
8 tbsp groundnut or vegetable oil
3 tbsp soy sauce (dark or light)
3–4 tbsp fresh lime juice
1 small head Romaine lettuce
1 small head red-leaf lettuce
1 head chicory (Belgian endive)
2½cm (1 in) piece fresh ginger, peeled and finely chopped
2 large cloves garlic, finely chopped
2–3 fresh jalapeño chilli peppers, finely chopped
2 tsp soft brown sugar
3 medium tomatoes, cut into fine wedges
2 spring onions, finely chopped
large handful of fresh coriander, roughly chopped

Place the steak strips in a large dish. Mix together
2 tablespoons of the oil, 2 tablespoons of the soy sauce

and 2 tablespoons of the lime juice in a small bowl. Pour over the meat, cover and leave in the fridge to marinate for at least 1 hour.

Tear the Romaine and red-leaf lettuce into bite-sized pieces. Divide the chicory into whole leaves and place in a plastic food bag with the lettuce. Set aside in the fridge until needed.

Meanwhile, in a blender or food processor, blend 3 tablespoons of the remaining oil with all the remaining soy sauce, all the remaining lime juice and the ginger, garlic, chilli peppers and brown sugar to make a dressing. Set on one side.

Heat a ridged frying pan or wok over a high heat until hot and add the remaining oil. Drain the steak, reserving the marinade, and add to the pan. Quickly stir-fry until the meat just starts to brown.

As soon as the steak is cooked, place the chilled salad leaves in a large serving bowl, toss over the tomato wedges, spring onions and chopped coriander and top with the freshly cooked steak strips. Quickly mix the reserved marinade into the prepared dressing, and pour this over the salad. Toss lightly to mix through and serve immediately.

Thai orange chicken salad
(Yam pew som)

Serves 4

Preparation and cooking time: 40–45 minutes

600g (1lb 5oz) chicken breast fillets, cut into thick
slices
6 tbsp coconut milk
2 tbsp Thai fish sauce
freshly ground black pepper
juice of 1 orange
½ tbsp light brown sugar
¼ tsp cayenne pepper
approximately 250–300g (8–10½oz) mixed salad
greens, enough to fill 4 large serving bowls
1 orange, peeled, pith removed and divided into
segments
1 fresh papaya, cut into thin strips
2 large handfuls fresh coriander, lightly chopped
handful fresh mint or basil leaves, lightly chopped
140g (5oz) unsalted cashew nuts
10 cherry tomatoes, sliced in half

Place the chicken slices in a large dish. In a small bowl,
mix together 3 tablespoons of the coconut milk and
1 tablespoon of the Thai fish sauce. Pour over the

chicken, mix well and leave to marinate in the fridge for at least 30 minutes.

Preheat the grill until hot. Place a generous sheet of foil on the grill pan or a roasting pan. Curl up the edges of the foil to prevent any juices from spilling over the sides. Remove the chicken strips from the marinade and lay out flat, in a single layer, on the foil (you can include some of the marinade). Sprinkle generously with black pepper. Place under the hot grill and cook the chicken for 5–7 minutes, turning once or twice, until it is cooked through and nicely browned. Remove from the heat and again sprinkle generously with pepper. Set aside and keep warm.

While the chicken is cooking, make a dressing by whisking together the orange juice, the remaining coconut milk and Thai fish sauce, the brown sugar and the cayenne pepper in a small bowl. Taste and add more sugar if necessary (the dressing should lean slightly towards the sweet side, as it will taste less sweet once it is on the salad).

Place the salad greens, orange segments, papaya strips, chopped fresh herbs, cashew nuts and cherry tomatoes in a large mixing bowl. Pour over half the dressing and toss well. Divide between four large serving bowls. Top each bowl with a quarter of the warm chicken strips. Drizzle over the remaining dressing and serve.

Spicy Thai prawn salad

Serves 4

Preparation and cooking time: 10 minutes

2 tbsp lime juice
4 tsp Thai fish sauce
1 tbsp rapeseed oil
2 tsp light brown sugar
½ tsp crushed chilli
450g (1lb) cooked and peeled small prawns
2–3 red, yellow or orange peppers, deseeded and thinly sliced
1 small cucumber, deseeded and thinly sliced
handful fresh mixed herbs, such as basil, coriander and mint, roughly chopped

Whisk the lime juice, fish sauce, rapeseed oil, brown sugar and crushed chilli together in a large serving bowl.

Add the prawns, sliced peppers, cucumber and fresh herbs. Toss to combine well and serve.

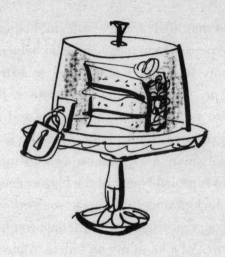

Acknowledgements

Joe

I don't want to come over all Oscars but I do owe some big thank yous to some people who have helped me along the way. Firstly I want to thank Roger Eric Smith, who will be the most surprised man on the planet when he discovers that I've managed to write and publish a book (with a little help obviously, but more of that shortly). I would also like to say an enormous heartfelt thanks to Joanne Spencer who has always been there for me and has had a huge role in helping me to become the person I am today and who helped me start and build my business. I must send an extra special thanks to my long-suffering big brother Fadi who ferried me to and from training sessions and sacrificed a lot of his personal life to help me make it as a professional sportsman. Also, grammy award winner David Arnold, who is probably one of the biggest geniuses I've ever been lucky enough to meet, you've been a real inspiration, a great friend and, whether you know it or not, the source of a lot of my best ideas. A big thanks to you all, you have all inspired me in different ways and without you none of this would have been possible.

I also want to say a big thanks to Jordan Paramor – without her patience and writing ability this would definitely not have been possible. And finally to all the team at Headline – Carly, Josh, Emily, Ruth, Sophie and everyone else who has worked on the book – you have been great ... if you guys can do this programme, anyone can!

Jordan

A huge thank you to Carla, Carly, Josh and Emily for all their amazing work on the book. Thanks to Mike for his support, and of course to fitness guru Joe. Mine's a champagne ...